The

BATCH
LADY

TO PETER, JAKE & ZARA
– THANK YOU FOR EVERYTHING.

HQ
An imprint of HarperCollinsPublishers Ltd
1 London Bridge Street
London SE1 9GF

10 9 8 7 6 5 4 3 2 1

First published in Great Britain by HQ
An imprint of HarperCollinsPublishers Ltd 2020

Text Copyright © Suzanne Mulholland 2020

Suzanne Mulholland asserts the moral right to be
identified as the author of this work. A catalogue
record for this book is available from the British
Library.

ISBN 978-0-00-837322-1

Our policy is to use papers that are natural, renewable
and recyclable products and made from wood grown
in sustainable forests. The logging and manufacturing
processes conform to the legal environmental
regulations of the country of origin.

For more information visit:
www.harpercollins.co.uk/green

Photography: Danielle Woods
Food styling: Rosie Ramsden
Prop styling: Linda Berlin and Wei Tang
Design & Art Direction: Georgina Hewitt
Editorial Director: Kate Fox
Project Editor: Daniel Hurst

Printed and bound by Rotolito (Italy)

Suzanne Mulholland

The

BATCH
LADY

SHOP ONCE. COOK ONCE.
EAT WELL ALL WEEK.

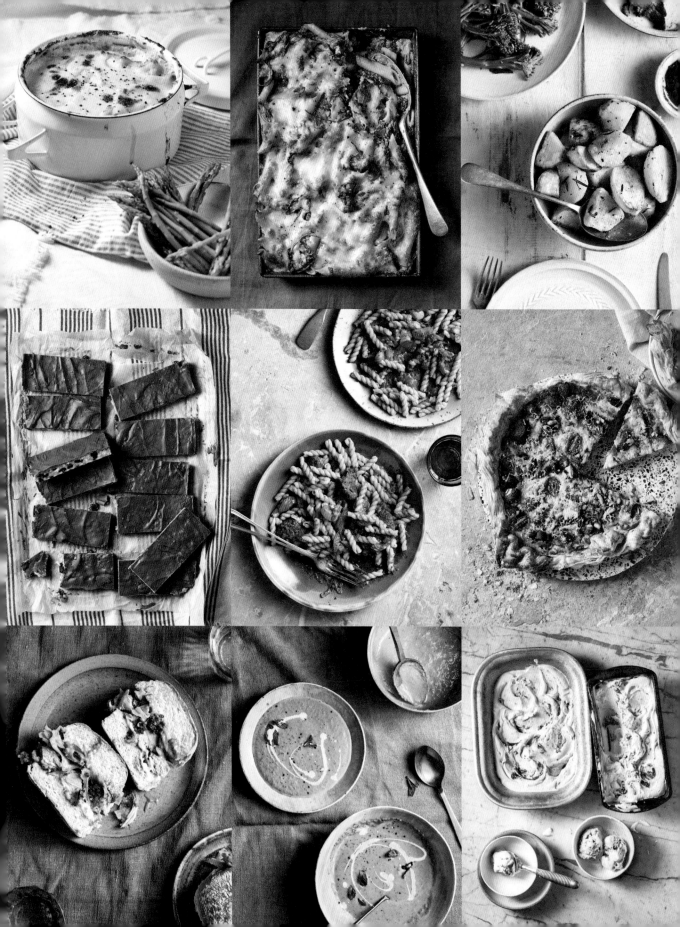

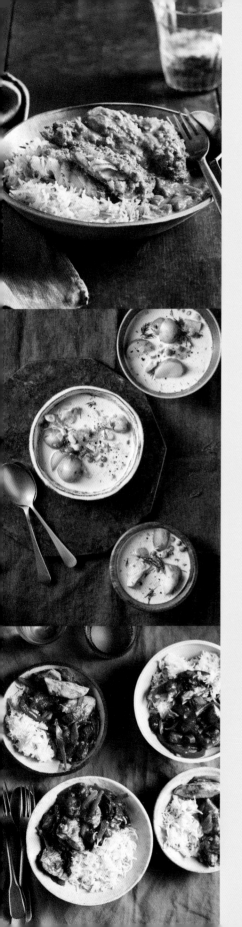

CONTENTS

WELCOME

My name is Suzanne Mulholland but you might know me as **The Batch Lady**.

Can I tell you a secret? I'm not a cook – far from it in fact. My transformation into The Batch Lady was not something I planned, but something that happened out of necessity.

As a busy wife and mother with a large extended family on my doorstep, I often felt like I was stuck in a kind of Groundhog Day – a slave to the kitchen who was forever trying to churn out tasty and nutritious meals night after night when, in truth, I would much rather be spending time with my kids or reading a good book. Add to this the fact that I live on a remote farm in the Scottish Borders with the nearest shop over 30 minutes' drive away and you'll start to get an idea of what a slog this could be. The worst thing was that I had always enjoyed cooking, but being chained to the kitchen day after day was starting to make me resent it. Something had to change. I had to get organized!

Luckily, organization is something I have been trained for. Literally. I had studied business and time management at university and have always used workarounds to get household chores done in the shortest possible time. With a new determination to apply these skills to mealtimes, I developed a system where I made batch-cooked meals in advance and stored them in the freezer. Soon, I was only cooking one day a week.

As time went on, I streamlined my system even further by pairing meals that had similar core ingredients together. This meant that I could, with careful planning and shopping, make multiple meals for the freezer at the same time. In no time at all, I found that I was able to reclaim time to spend doing the things I loved, with the added bonuses that we were also eating better, saving money and had very little food waste.

Liberated from the kitchen, friends soon began to notice how carefree and organized I was at mealtimes, so I started sharing some of my hacks with them. In no time at all, word had got out and people were asking for more tips and tricks, curious to see if they could use the same techniques in their own homes. I invited twenty curious friends around to my house and gave them a live demonstration of how to cook 10 meals in 1 hour. My guests were blown away by the demo and encouraged me to share a video of the event on YouTube and Facebook. The Batch Lady was born!

Looking back, it's ironic that something that I started to save myself time has now become my full-time job! Standing in front of that group of friends in my kitchen I would never have believed that my message would resonate with so many people but, just two years later, I have been lucky enough to share my message with thousands of people through my website and social media channels, and now this book!

As our lives get ever busier, it can be harder and harder to find time for the things that really count. I hope that the tips, tricks and recipes in these pages can help you reclaim your time, alleviate your stress and fill the tables and bellies of you and your loved ones with tasty, home-cooked food.

Believe in the batch!

Suzanne

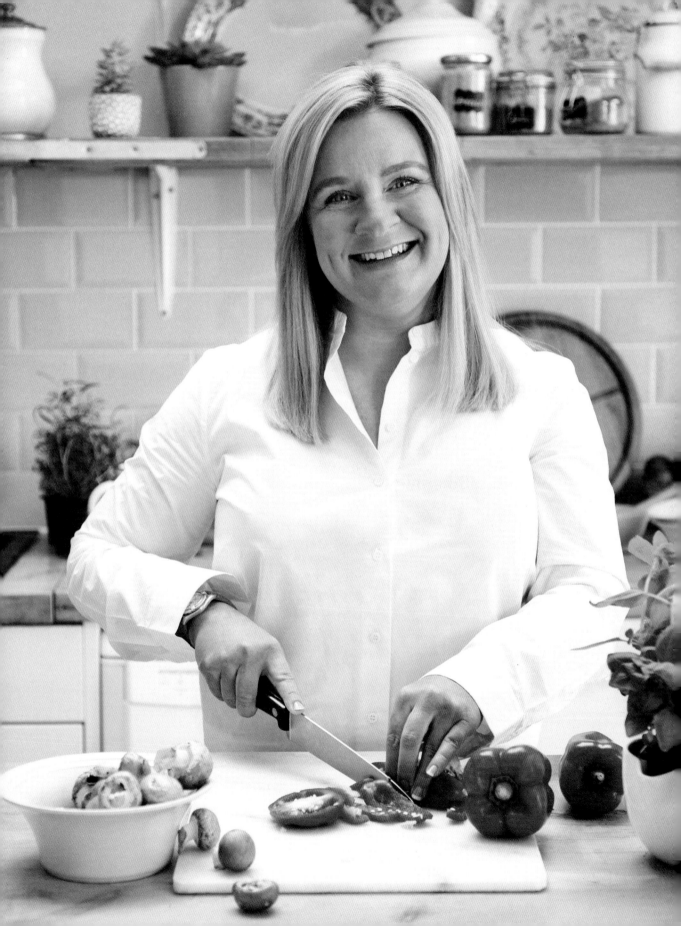

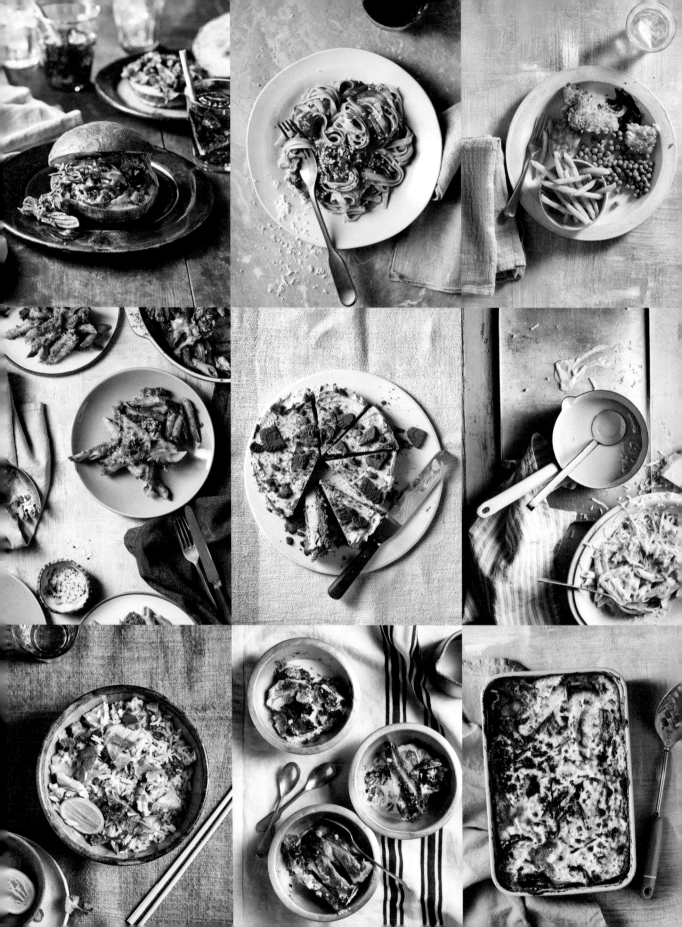

INTRODUCTION

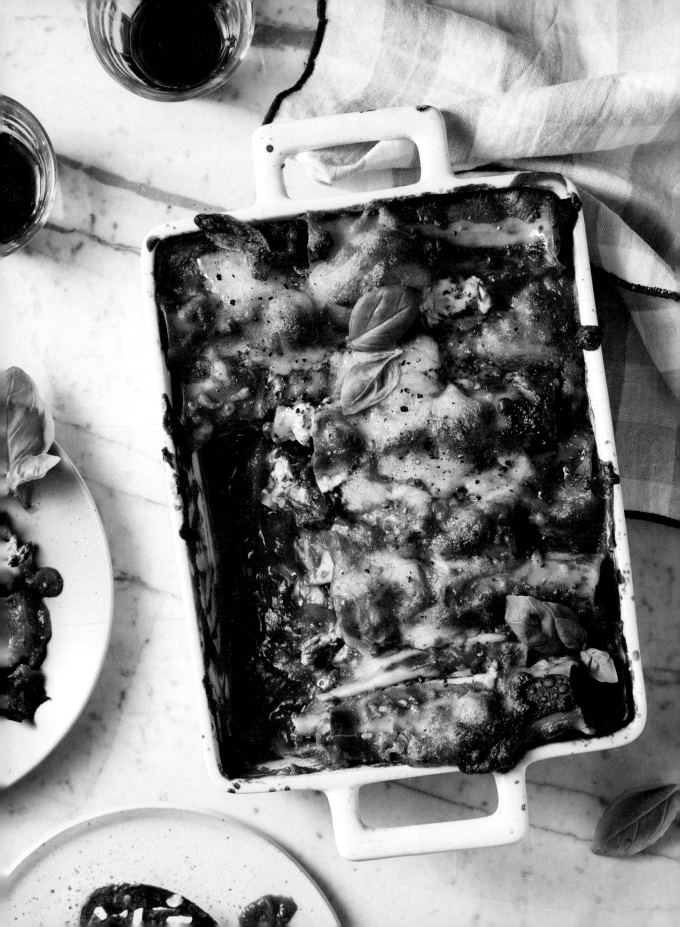

WHAT IS BATCHING?

To a lot of people, batching meals can seem complicated at first, but it is actually a far simpler way of cooking. With a little bit of planning, you can save yourself time and money every week, allowing you to spend more of your time on the things you enjoy. Here's how ...

BRINGING TIME MANAGEMENT HOME

On the surface, the phrase 'time management' sounds very impersonal and businesslike, and not at all like something that you want to worry about in your lovely, cozy home. In fact, the whole point of introducing this technique at home is to make more time for the fun stuff. Freeing you up to spend more time playing with the kids, more time snuggling up with a glass of wine and a good book, more time spent with friends and family. It's about giving yourself time to exhale and process, and in today's relentlessly busy world, that can only be a good thing. In practice, time management is simply looking at the many tasks that take up your time and working out how they can be streamlined to free you up for other stuff. The stuff that matters.

This method can be applied to everything from the way you get dressed in the morning, how you organize your laundry or do the housework to what you are making for dinner in the evening. Streamlining my life like this has saved my sanity and allowed me time to feel like me again – rather than some kind of cooking and cleaning automaton!

I apply this approach to every aspect of my life but the thing that has made the biggest difference, by far, is time managing the food that I cook for my family on a daily basis. Something that used to dominate every evening can now be accomplished in just an hour a week. Cooking in this way has allowed me to reclaim my evenings and my enjoyment of cooking – and it can do the same for you!

HEADSPACE NOT PERFECTIONISM

Batching is not about perfectionism. It's about **headspace**.

I get asked by people all the time if I'm a perfectionist, to which I usually respond with a burst of laughter, because I am far from this. Being organized and managing my time is not

about everything being perfect, it's about giving myself a break from constantly thinking about those chores that have to be done day after day. Instead, my week is planned and I feel freer to enjoy the fun things, like spending time with my family and friends.

THE BENEFITS OF BATCHING

Batch cooking isn't just about saving time in the kitchen – it also saves time on all the related chores like planning, shopping and washing up, too.

How many of us get to three in the afternoon and start to panic about what we're going to have for dinner that evening? We swing by the supermarket on the way home and browse the shelves for inspiration, torn between the convenience of a pizza or ready meal and the pressure we feel to put something homemade and nutritious on the table.

My way of cooking does away with this stress. With a little planning, you can streamline your shopping so that you can buy all the food for the week in one go. All of the planning is done in advance, so your daily mental load is lightened and you are only buying the food that you really need, meaning that there is no waste, all of which is far better for you, your wallet and the environment!

When it comes to cooking, you can pretty much batch anything – if I'm going to be making a mess in the kitchen, I'd rather make five meals at once and have one big mess to tidy up as opposed to having to clean down the kitchen every night of the week. If the recipes are made using a lot of the same ingredients and techniques, all the better.

The old-fashioned image of batch cooking is often centered around creating a huge vat of one meal, say a large pot of soup or a huge curry that you will be eating for weeks, but, for me, batch cooking is about cooking food that uses similar ingredients to create very different meals. For example, in one batch you can create a Moussaka (p.86) and some Lamb & Feta Burgers (p.87), or even a Potato Dauphinoise (p.196) and a Spanish Omelette (p.197) – recipes that use many of the same ingredients, but offer great variety in your weekly meal plan.

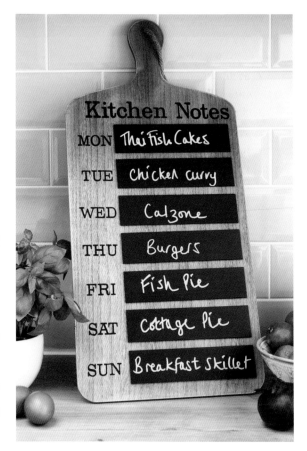

Kitchen Notes

MON — Thai Fish Cakes
TUE — Chicken curry
WED — Calzone
THU — Burgers
FRI — Fish Pie
SAT — Cottage Pie
SUN — Breakfast Skillet

THE BATCH METHOD

The recipes in this book are all for fuss-free midweek meals. Nothing fancy or unachievable, just real food for the way real people cook, every day.

When planning the food for this book, I put a post on my social media channels asking for my followers to share their weekly meal planners with me. What quickly became very clear was that people were looking for simple food that tasted great and could be prepared with minimum fuss. With that in mind, I planned the recipes in this book around family favourites that, with a little batching magic, can be on the table in a jiffy.

Each recipe is pared back to its basics – this will save you time and, I promise, I have only cut corners where it doesn't impact on the final result.

If you are cooking for a special occasion or just want to dress up your dinner a bit, I've suggested some ways you can zhuzh (my favourite word!) up some of the recipes, and you'll see these marked on the pages as you work your way through.

If a meal contains spices, I have erred on the side of caution and opted for delicate rather than 'blow-your-head-off' hot, as my meals are designed to be family friendly. If you like more spice, simply adjust the levels to your tastes. As a general rule, it's good to remember that spice can always be added, but never removed!

WORKING IN PAIRS

All of the recipes in this book are paired-up with another. These are dishes that lend themselves to being prepared together, and throughout the recipe methods you will find tips on how to save time by jumping between the two. Sound complicated? I promise you it's not! Each of the meals can also be made as a standalone dish, serving 4–6 people, so it's up to you if you want to batch it with the other meal.

Once you've got the hang of batching two recipes together, you can start doubling up and making four full meals at once!

ODD ONES OUT

When pairing recipes, it sometimes makes sense to match a savoury dish with a sweet, or a meat dish with a veggie. If you take my Plait recipes (p.74–75) as an example, you'll see that both recipes use the same technique, which is why they are paired together, but this does mean that you'll find a sweet recipe in the middle of the meat chapter! To help you identify this, all of the recipes are colour-coded and marked with a symbol in the top corner so that you know exactly what kind of recipe you are looking at. The symbols are:

P POULTRY

F FISH

S SIDES & SAUCES

M MEAT

V VEG

D DESSERTS

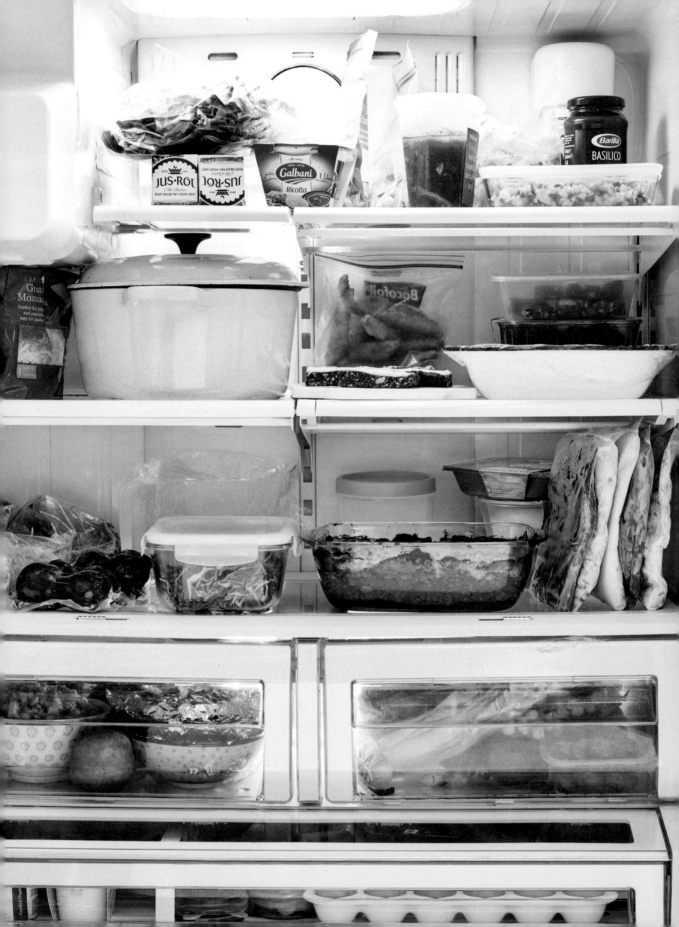

TO COOK. TO FREEZE. TO COOK FROM FROZEN

Every dish in this book can be cooked fresh, or made in advance and stored in the freezer until needed. At the bottom of each recipe you will see the headings 'To Cook', 'To Freeze' and 'To Cook from Frozen', so all you need to do is follow the instructions according to how you want to prepare the meal. Simple!

Some meals can be cooked directly from frozen and others need to be defrosted first. Full instructions on the various ways of defrosting meals can be found on page 30, but the simplest way is simply to transfer it from the freezer to the fridge the evening before you want to serve it and leave to defrost slowly overnight.

NO-COOK MEALS

Throughout this book you will see no-cook meals – these are meals that are assembled from entirely uncooked or frozen ingredients and then stored in bags in the freezer until needed. No cooking required! (At least until the day you want to serve them.)

The benefit of these meals is that they take very little time to prepare and freeze. Preparing the food in this way also means that when you take the bag out of the freezer, the food is being cooked for the first time – great for things like fish and chicken that can dry out when reheated.

I often pair a no-cook meal with a cooked meal, as you can easily prepare your no-cook meal while your other recipe is bubbling away on the stove or baking in the oven. For example, while your Luxury Seafood Chowder (p.122) is simmering away, you can spend 10 minutes assembling a no-cook Easy-but-Luxury Fish Pie (p.122) to pop straight in the freezer. The two dishes use similar ingredients, so the extra prep is minimal, and you have created two full meals in the same time it would have taken to make just the chowder alone.

THREE WAYS WITH…

Within the recipe chapters you'll see features titled 'Three Ways With …' – these pages show you how, with a little bit of additional prep, one meal can be served in three different ways. There are some recipes that lend themselves particularly well to this treatment, and in each chapter throughout the book you'll find a few. A great example of this is my recipe for Pulled Pork on page 92. Cooking one large shoulder of pork will yield enough meat for several meals, so it's nice to have different options for how to serve it. On pages 94–95 you'll see that one delicious batch of Pulled Pork can be mixed with sweetcorn, spring onions and cheese

and used as a delicious topping for baked sweet potatoes, spooned into fluffy brioche buns and served with a topping of apple sauce and crunchy fresh apple or spiced up with jalapenos and used as a delicious filling for quesadillas.

The recipes for sauces in the Sides & Sauces chapter (p.184–225) are another example of where this feature is used, as once you've made your Basic Tomato Sauce, Pesto or Enchilada Pasta Sauce, it's useful to have a variety of options on how to use them. In this way you'll be able to use the recipes in this book time and again and they'll feel fresh and different every time.

10 MEALS IN 1 HOUR

Are you ready to move to ultimate batcher status? Once you are used to using the paired-up recipes and doubling up on ingredients, the next stage is to move on to making even more meals with similar ingredients all at the same time.

At the end of every recipe chapter you will find a special section on how to cook 10 meals in 1 hour. The only exceptions to this are the Sides & Sauces and Desserts chapters – mainly because I couldn't be trusted to have 10 desserts at once!

Though it sounds like an impossible task, once you've got the hang of cooking this way, you'll never go back. And I'll tell you a secret, it's actually pretty simple! With a little organization, you will be amazed how many family meals you can make in such a short space of time.

The meals in these sections are all made using similar base ingredients, so you probably won't

want to eat them every night in succession, but if you put two in the fridge for the week ahead and the rest in the freezer, you'll be well stocked with tasty meals that are a ready to go at a moment's notice – and all with just 1 hour's investment of your time!

Here's how it works: In each of the four sections (Poultry, Meat, Fish and Veg), I give you a list of ingredients for each recipe, a full shopping list for the entire batch and one long method to make the five meals, each one scaled up to serve eight people.

This means that at the end of the hour you will have a double portion of each of the five meals ready to be portioned up and frozen for later. That's a total of 40 individual servings made in 1 hour! Below are some tips to get you started ...

SHOPPING FOR INGREDIENTS

Once you have decided which of the 10-meals sections you want to cook from, simply check the shopping list for the entire batch against what you already have in your cupboards.

If I'm planning to cook one of these menus, I will often do an online shop and have it delivered

just before I want to start cooking. That way, I can simply arrange everything on my sides ready to go without having to put it all away first then having to dig through my kitchen to extract it all again later.

PREPPING YOUR KITCHEN

Before you embark on one of these mammoth cook-offs, you will want to make sure that your kitchen is clean and that your countertops are clear to arrange your ingredients on. It's a good idea to make sure your food-waste and recycling bins are empty as well as your dishwasher, if you

have one – that way you can tidy as you go. I also fill my sink with hot, soapy water so I can quickly wash my utensils as I use them, ready for reusing. I find it helps to have kitchen cleaner and fresh tea towels on hand so that I can quickly wash down the sides as I hop between prepping meals.

This also avoids having a huge mound of washing up to tackle at the end!

Once your kitchen is ready to go, it's a good idea to lay out all of the equipment that you will need – that way you won't be scrabbling through the cupboards trying to find a pan or utensil halfway through a recipe. Don't forget to have a supply of freezer bags and a pen for labelling to hand, too, so that you can bag up your wares ready for freezing at the end of each recipe.

SETTING OUT YOUR INGREDIENTS

In each 10-meals section, you will find an individual list of ingredients for each of the recipes you will be making, in the order that you will be making them. Make clearly-defined piles of ingredients according to each of these lists, that way you can easily jump back and forth between each recipe without wondering which pile of onions is for which recipe! If you have the space, leave the work surface directly around your stovetop clear to use during the actual cooking, then set the piles of ingredients out so that the pile closest to you is for the first recipe that you will be making, and so on.

BE REALISTIC WITH YOUR TIME

Don't be disheartened if it takes more than an hour the first time you attempt to make one of these menus. Like anything new, it can take a little practice to get the hang of but, believe me, once you're in the swing of it, each time will be quicker. Because I have made them so many times, I can now cook some of the menus in just 30 minutes!

A top tip for cooking these menus is to choose a time when the house is quiet and you won't get distracted. When my kids were small, I would batch when they were at nursery, now they are teenagers and sleep late on Sunday mornings, I now batch for the week ahead then.

FILLING YOUR FREEZER

If you want a variety of dishes in your freezer and prefer not to cook from scratch at all mid week, then I suggest cooking one of these 10-meals sections every few weeks. I make a 10-meal batch every second Sunday, and if I cooked the fish batch last time, then I will do the chicken batch next. That way, I always have variety of different foods in my freezer.

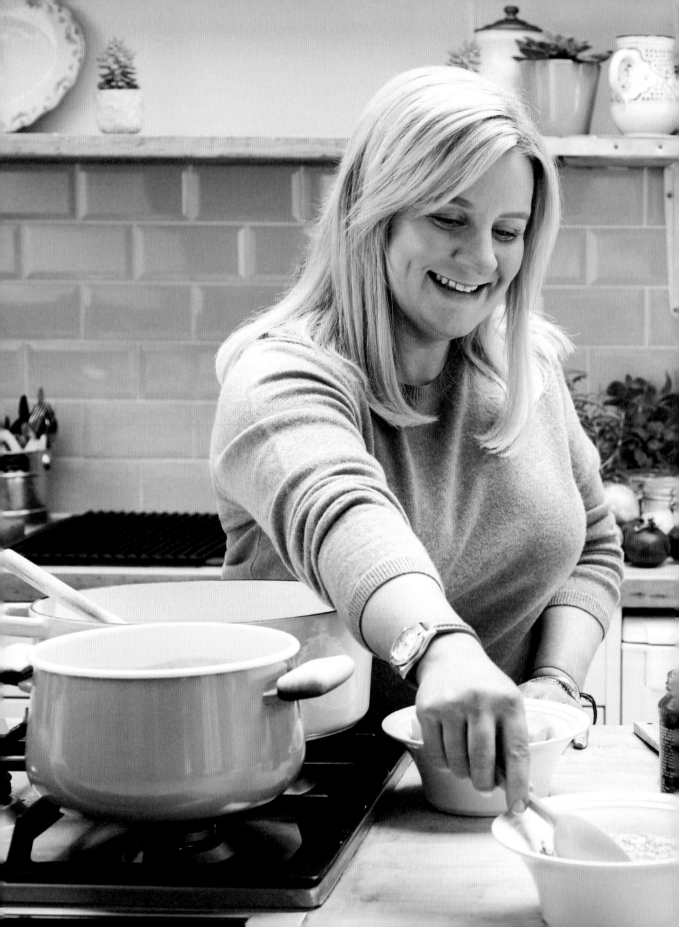

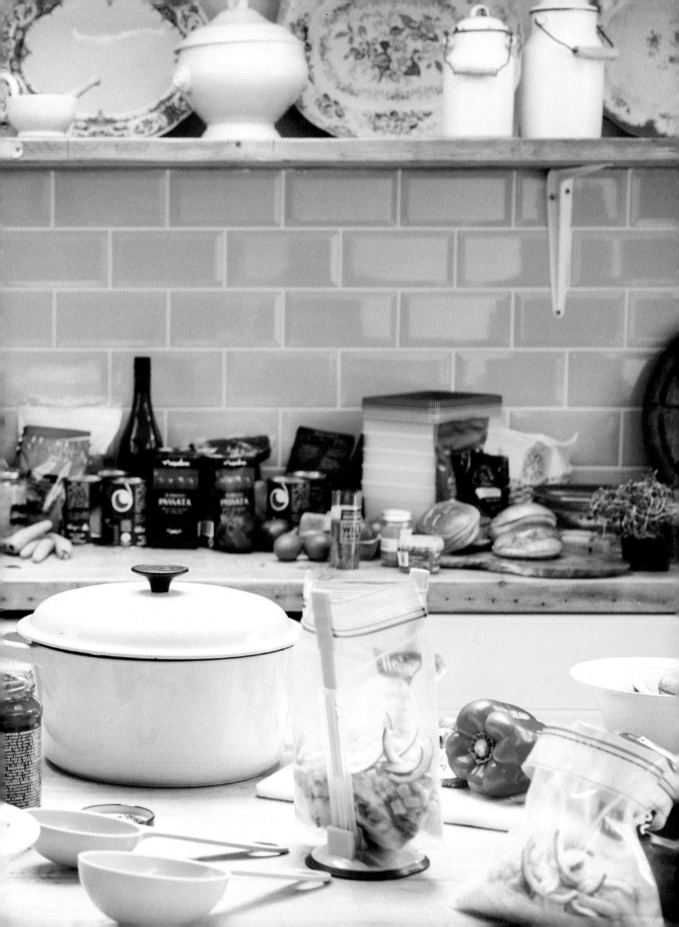

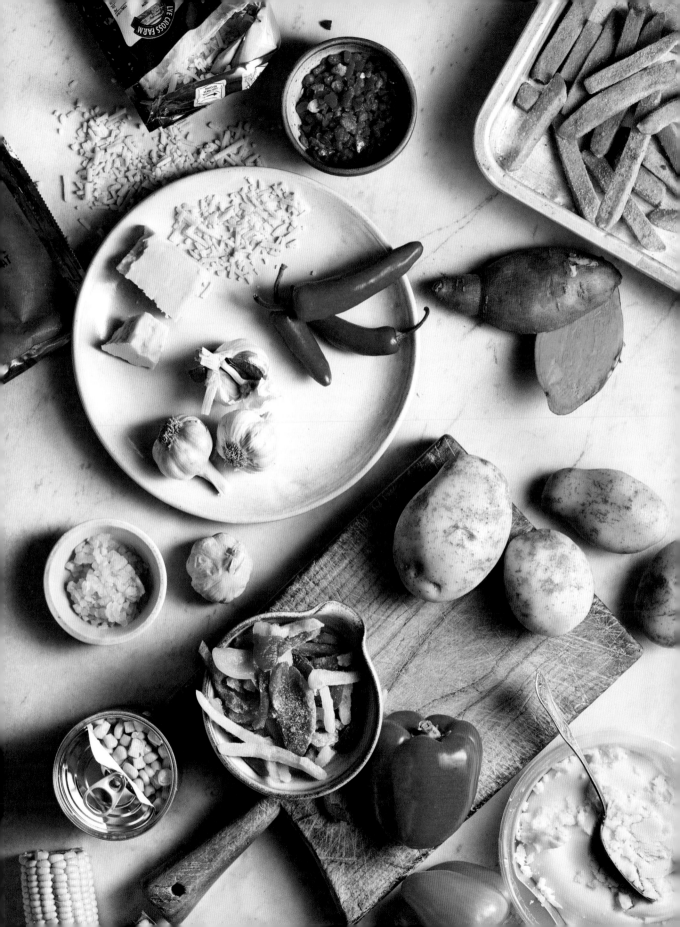

THE BATCH LADY LARDER

You will notice as you go through this book that I use many different ingredients, from ready-made, shop-bought mash to frozen veg and herbs. I'm all about time saving so I want the fastest way to make a meal – if it requires something shop bought, then so be it. I figure that my made-in-advance, home-cooked meal with the odd shop-bought ingredient is much better than me not cooking at all.

EASY CHEATS

'Cheats', as I like to call them, are my saving grace. I'm a big believer that experts generally know best. If my dishwasher is broken then I call a plumber – I would never attempt to fix it myself! The same applies if I need to use pastry in a recipe – I leave it to the experts and simply buy the ready-rolled variety. It saves me time and stress. It's quicker, I know the recipe will work and I won't waste any ingredients. (Besides, I'm rubbish at pastry!)

That said, I'm a no judgment type of gal. If you want to make your own mash or pastry, then by all means go ahead. If you prefer to chop fresh onions instead of buying frozen, then do. Just remember that it will take longer to make the recipe than it would if you used the 'cheats' listed.

PASTES
I tend not to use many jarred sauces, but I do love concentrated pastes as they really pack a punch of flavour, especially curry pastes. When I am feeding my family, it's really important that the meals I serve taste the same every time that I make them – kids really notice if a recipe is different from the last time – and pastes are brilliant for this. I'm not an expert in Thai or Japanese cuisine, and this is another example of a time that I would rather leave it to the professionals! From a health standpoint, concentrated pastes are generally a lot better to use than large jars of ready-made sauces, which can have lots of hidden sugars.

CHOPPED, FROZEN VEGETABLES
I'm a huge advocate of pre-chopped, frozen vegetables for many reasons. Obviously, they save a lot of time as someone else has done the hard work for you but they are also usually packed and flash frozen within an hour of being picked, so they retain all their healthy nutrients. They are also often cheaper than fresh, which, given the work that has already been done for you, still astounds me. They will keep in the freezer for ages, so you don't have to worry about using up the veg languishing in the back of the veg drawer and you always have a ready supply on hand.

The one downside is that they come in plastic packaging, but many fresh vegetables nowadays do too. The good news is that the frozen-food industry has pledged to go plastic-free and is looking to change packaging.

The only two vegetables that I prefer to use fresh are broccoli and mushrooms, as they just don't freeze well. Otherwise, I'm a freezer fan all the way!

If you prefer to use fresh veg, then go ahead – just be aware that the meals will take longer to prepare because of the extra chopping and peeling involved.

CHOPPED, FROZEN HERBS

Fresh herbs are so lovely, but they're expensive and have a short shelf-life. Because of this, I always have a ready supply of frozen herbs in my freezer which are cheaper than fresh and keep for as long as you need them. Most supermarkets have a good range of frozen herbs but, if you can't find them where you live, just substitute them for fresh or dried.

READY-MADE MASH

This is my biggest time-saver of all, and I have to say I'm a huge fan! Ready-made mash isn't just convenient, it also freezes far better than homemade, which has a tendency to separate and become watery in the freezer. Store-bought, ready-made mash has been made in a large churner, so tends to keep its lovely, fluffy texture once frozen and defrosted.

READY-ROLLED PASTRY

Ready-rolled pastry is a great time saver and, most importantly, it always works! It also freezes really well. If I'm making a chicken pie, for example, I simply freeze the pie filling alongside a roll of puff pastry, then reheat the filling in the oven, with squares of puff pastry alongside. Everyone gets a spoonful of pie filling crowned with a beautifully puffed, golden square of puff pastry. All the joy of a pie without any of the hassle!

READY-ROLLED PIZZA DOUGH

Shop-bought pizzas are expensive and often disappointing. Making your own at home is easy, fun for the kids and you have complete control over the toppings! I use packs of ready-rolled pizza dough, which are great for making pizzas and also my Calzone recipes (p.82–83).

STORECUPBOARD INGREDIENTS

As well as the 'cheats' that I always fall back on, I always keep my cupboards stocked with a few essential ingredients that are versatile, store well and are packed with flavour.

DRIED HERBS AND SPICES

Jars of dried Italian seasoning, mixed herbs or oregano are great to have on hand. I use these in a lot of my recipes, so it's good to get the large jars if possible. I also use a lot of fajita or taco seasoning to add instant spice to any Mexican or Cajun-inspired dishes, such as the Cajun Pork Steaks on page 47. You can buy the seasoning in individual sachets or jars and it's a good idea to stock up on a few so that you always have a ready supply on hand.

STORECUPBOARD SUNDRIES

The other essentials that pack a lot of bang for their buck and, therefore, crop up a lot in my recipes are Worcestershire sauce, olive oil, tinned tomatoes, passata and condensed soup.

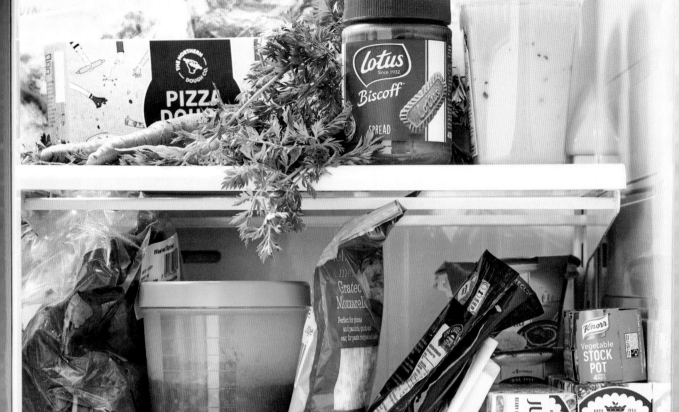
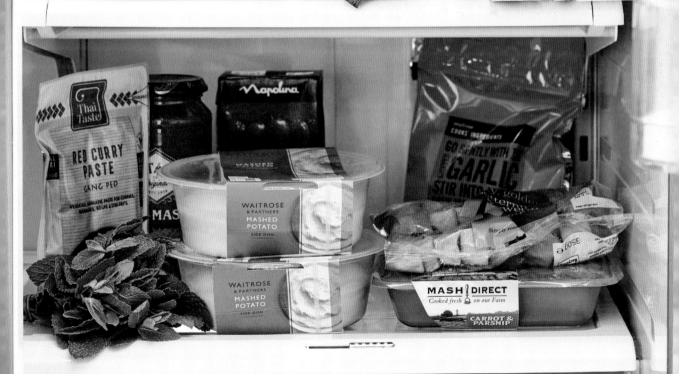

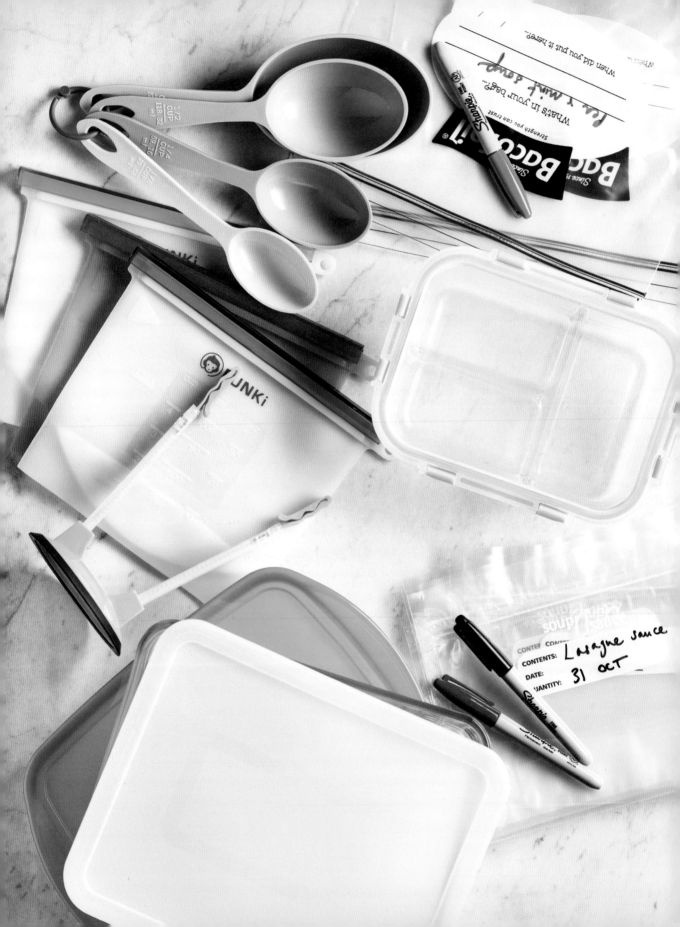

ESSENTIAL KIT

As you work through the recipes in this book, you will see that there are certain tools that are used time and again to speed up the batching process. In truth, there are only a couple of things that are really essential, but it is worth investing if you are going to be adopting this way of cooking.

MEASURING CUPS

Cups are a brilliant time-saver as they save all the time spent painstakingly weighing your ingredients. Instead, you can simply scoop the ingredients into the right-sized cup and pop it straight into your dish. I have listed cup measurements first in all of my recipes (though there are of course gram measurements, too), to try and get you into this way of thinking. It's important to be aware that 1 cup is a standard measurement, so don't just grab the mug that you make your morning coffee in! What you really need is a set of **large measuring spoons in cup sizes.** They are available from my website (details on p.247) and other retailers. For more information on using cups, see page 31.

FREEZER BAGS

Freezer bags are great space savers, as you can freeze everything flat and thus get more in. They also prevent freezer burn as you can take all the excess air out of the bag before sealing. Lastly, they help food defrost quicker as they are thin and flat, so you don't end up with a huge block to defrost as you would do using a tub. Most brands are now washable and reusable so no need to feel bad about using too much plastic!

MARKER PENS

Great for writing on your bags and won't rub off in the freezer, so you never end up with a UFO (Unidentified Frozen Object!) Ensure you label everything as it all looks the same once frozen.

TWO LARGE COOKING POTS

'Go big or go home' is a saying that comes to mind. You will need some large pots and, if you're going to invest in anything for batching, I'd say good, stainless steel pots that can go from your stove top to oven should be at the top of your list!

TWO LARGE BOWLS

Much like the pots, these are good to have, and will be used throughout most of these recipes.

GLASS DISHES WITH PLASTIC LIDS

I cannot recommend these highly enough, they transition from freezer to oven perfectly – just take the lid off and pop it straight in the oven. They also look good so you can put them in the middle of the table and serve your meals straight from the dish. I use these when I am batching fish pies, enchiladas, pasta bakes etc. I recommend Pyrex dishes as the best for freezing.

Finally, the following kitchen items are always good to have on hand: knifes, chopping boards, foil, Tupperware, scissors. If you get into batching and are using freezer bags a lot, then I would also recommend a set of 'baggy holders' that help hold your bags open. These are available from my website and other online retailers.

GET ORGANIZED!

Planning what you are going to eat during the week ahead may seem laborious, but it saves time, money and waste, and often means that you eat a greater variety of food and that that food is more healthy. In fact, planning and writing down the meals that you want to make means you are much more likely to actually make those meals. Writing a meal plan can be daunting and many people struggle for inspiration the first few times, so below are some tips to help you get started.

HOW TO MEAL PLAN

There are many different ways to write your meal plan, from physical boards that hang in your kitchen to apps that you can carry with you on your phone. I like to use an old-fashioned board, however, as it helps me to have my list of meals for the week ahead hanging in my kitchen. This also means that the family knows what they will be eating ahead of time, which helps avoid mutterings of dissent if they're surprised with a meal that's not their favourite!

When starting to write my meal plan, I look at my diary for the week and work the plan around that. If I know that I'll be ferrying the kids around to various afterschool activities on Tuesday, then I'll make sure to plan something quick and easy for then. If I'm in the house all day on Thursday, but tied up with work, I'll plan something that I can pop in the oven and forget about for a few hours. I like to start by thinking about which proteins we will be eating throughout the week to ensure they are varied. An example week might look like this:

Monday: Meat-free
Tuesday: Beef
Wednesday: Fish
Thursday: Chicken
Friday: Fakeaway

Once I know my schedule and have the basic outline of which proteins we will be eating on each day, I start to think about the specific meals that I will cook. So, following the breakdown that I have outlined above, the weekly menu might look like:

Monday: Spanish Omelette
Tuesday: Shepherd's Pie
Wednesday: Thai Sweet Potato Fishcakes
Thursday: Spinach & Ricotta Stuffed Chicken
Friday: Calzone

If you are vegetarian, I would suggest taking a similar approach to ensure that you are eating a variety of foods throughout the week. Plan your menu so that you are focusing on one main ingredient, such as potatoes, beans or pulses, on each night, then add in the usual Friday-night curry or fakeaway. A well-balanced weekly vegetarian meal plan might look like this:

Monday: Baked Spinach Ziti
Tuesday: Chilli Bean Burgers
Wednesday: Spanish Omelette
Thursday: Oven-baked Mushroom Risotto
Friday: Thai Red Sweet Potato Curry

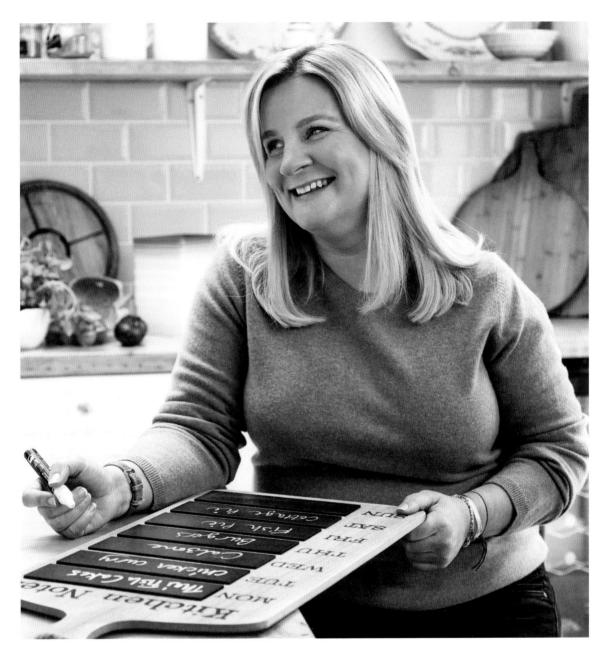

PLANNING FIVE DAYS OUT OF SEVEN

You will notice that I only ever plan my meals Monday–Friday. This is because, no matter how well you plan, there are always hiccups along the way and plans inevitably change throughout the week, meaning that food could potentially be wasted. By building in a two-day buffer, you can swap one or two of the meals to the weekend without wasting any food. If everything goes to plan, then then weekends are generally the time when you have a bit more time in the kitchen to cook something from scratch, or might eat out, so this gives you the freedom to still do that.

HOW TO USE YOUR FREEZER

Your freezer is the kitchen equivalent of an on-demand TV. Nowadays, very few people will sit down and watch their favourite show at the time it is airing – we record it or watch it on catch-up at a time that suits us. Used properly, your freezer can do just the same for your food, meaning that you can make your meals ahead of time then pull them out and defrost them later at a time that suits you.

NOTES ON FOOD SAFETY

Your freezer should not be the place where old leftovers go to live until you finally throw them out. You want to make sure than you are using what you freeze and constantly refreshing your freezer with fresh, in-date food.

When you batch cook it's important to maintain good kitchen hygiene at all times to help reduce the transfer of bacteria. This is simple to do, just make sure that your surfaces are cleaned with antibacterial spray before you start and always be aware of what you are touching,

ensuring that you wash your hands thoroughly between touching raw and cooked foods.

Always do a quick clear up of utensils, pots and pans as you finish each recipe, making sure to also spray and wipe clean your surfaces – this is not only important from a hygiene point of view, it will also make the end clean down much quicker!

When working with chicken, do not rinse it first. Washing chicken in your home can easily spread bacteria. Simply use the chicken straight from the packet.

TIPS ON FREEZING

Always leave food to cool to room temperature before packaging to freeze. Wrapping your food in clingfilm and foil, or storing in freezer bags, reduces the chance of freezer burn.

If you are using glass dishes or plastic tubs, try to fill them to the top, leaving a small space for expansion – using a dish that is too big will leave the food exposed to air, causing freezer burn.

When packaging anything for the freezer, it is vital that it is labelled with the recipe name, the date and whether the food is raw or cooked. I also add cooking instructions to my labels so that I can refer to the label after defrosting my food.

It is important to freeze meals fast, as food starts to deteriorate the second it is made. As soon as a meal has cooled, package it up and transfer to the freezer. If you are freezing flat in freezer bags, try not to pile up lots of unfrozen meals on top of each other as this will prevent air from circulating and they will take longer to freeze. You can pile them up once they're frozen.

If you are scaling a recipe up, freeze the food in multiple batches. This means that you can remove the meals from the freezer a portion at a time. Large batches take much longer to defrost and can result in food wastage.

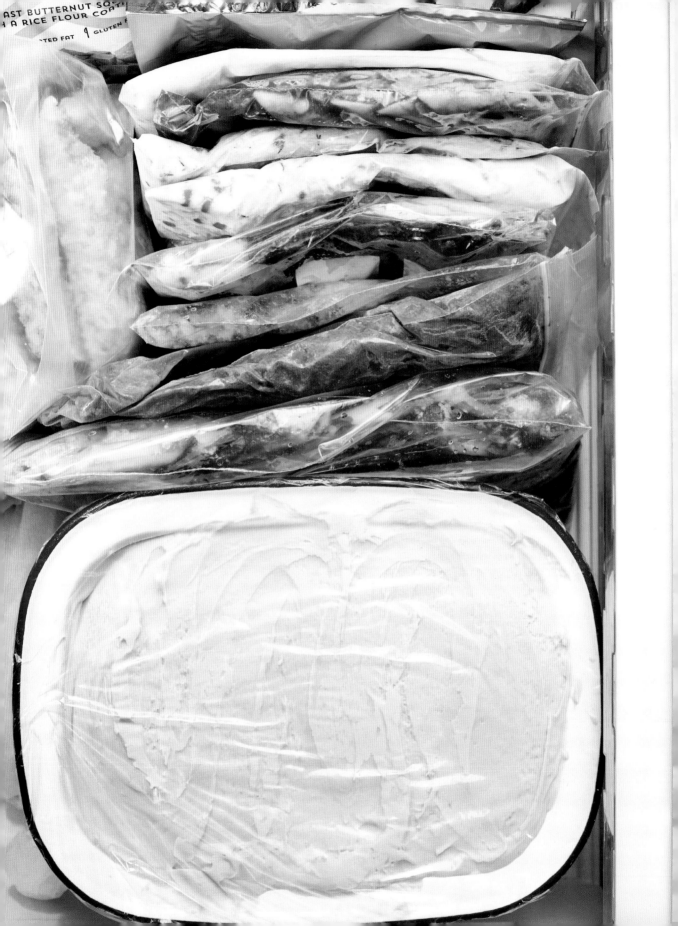

TIPS ON DEFROSTING

Many meals in this book can be cooked from frozen – just check the bottom of each recipe for instructions, though in general it will take 50 per cent longer than cooking from defrosted.

As a rule, I don't cook chicken from frozen. From a safety standpoint, raw chicken should not be cooked from frozen at all. Chicken that has been frozen cooked can, in theory, be safely cooked from frozen, but I still prefer to defrost it first and make sure it's piping hot before serving, and advise you to do the same.

There are three main ways to defrost food:

IN THE FRIDGE

Current guidelines recommend defrosting food in the fridge overnight. It is best to put thawing food in a dish to catch any water run-off. Defrosting in your fridge can take a long time, especially if you have frozen something in a large container. With this in mind, I like to combine this way with the water method, below.

IN COLD WATER

Make sure that the container your frozen food is stored in is watertight, then place it in a basin of cold water (never use hot!) Doing this speeds up the defrosting process. And makes for a very quick defrost if you have frozen meals flat in freezer bags.

IN THE MICROWAVE

Most microwaves have specific defrosting programmes, so just follow the manufacturers' instructions for your specific brand, remembering to stir your food a few times as it defrosts.

TAKING THINGS OUT OF THE FREEZER

I get so many messages from people asking how I remember to remove meals from the freezer. The secret is to make it a regular part of your daily routine. I set a reminder alarm on my phone that goes off at 6pm (the time that I serve dinner every evening) – I'm in the kitchen anyway, so I simply grab the next night's meal out of the freezer when the alarm goes off.

STORING MEALS IN THE FRIDGE

Once cooked, most meals will last for 3–4 days in the fridge, so, if batching at the weekend, you can keep the meals for the first half of the week in the fridge, then freeze the remainder.

If you have defrosted a meal you should eat it within 24 hours of it being fully defrosted

SMALL FREEZER STORAGE

You can still batch cook even with a small freezer! If you're challenged for space, I suggest freezing meals flat in bags, you may have to fold the bag over slightly to get it to fit into the drawer space, but you can store a lot of bags in this way. In a three-drawer freezer, I keep one drawer for frozen veg and herbs (and ice cream!), then the other two drawers are free to fill with batched meals.

USING CUPS

Throughout this book you will see that the measurements for ingredients are listed in cups first. I use cups for one reason only – they make cooking faster! They can also be used for stirring and even serving up a meal. I have also included gram and millimetre measurements in my ingredients lists, but for reference volume equivalents for cups are listed, right:

- 1 cup/240ml/16 tablespoons
- ¾ cup/180ml/12 tablespoons
- ⅔ cup/160ml/11 tablespoons
- ½ cup/120ml/8 tablespoons
- ⅓ cup/80ml/5½ tablespoons
- ¼ cup/60ml/4 tablespoons

PORTIONING MEALS WITH CUPS

Doubling or tripling a recipe is a great way of working when you are batch cooking, and is something I recommend, but, when faced with an enormous vat of food, it can be difficult to gauge how many people it will actually serve.

Using measuring cups to portion out meals can help with this. The general rule is that one level cup of scoopable food (Bolognese/curry/stew etc.) will feed one adult, whereas half a cup should be enough to feed a child under 10 years old.

FROZEN VERSUS FRESH

As I covered earlier in the introduction, I am a big fan of 'cheat' ingredients to save on time. My most commonly used are frozen onions, garlic, sliced peppers and spinach. If you would rather use fresh, simply use the chart below to work out how much of each ingredient you will need.

Frozen Ingredient	Amount	Fresh Equivalent
Frozen, chopped onions	1 cup	1 onion, finely chopped
Frozen, chopped red onions	1 cup	1 red onion, finely chopped
Frozen, chopped garlic	1 tsp	1 clove, crushed
Frozen, sliced peppers	1 cup	1 pepper, sliced
Frozen, chopped spinach	2 cubes	½ bag fresh spinach
Frozen, sliced carrots	1 cup	2 carrots, sliced

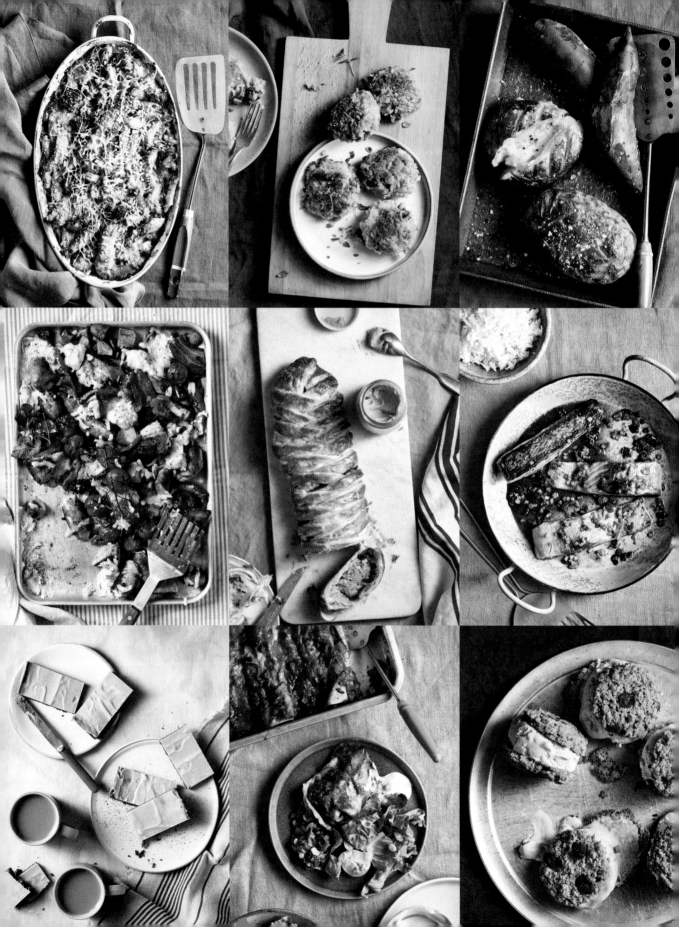

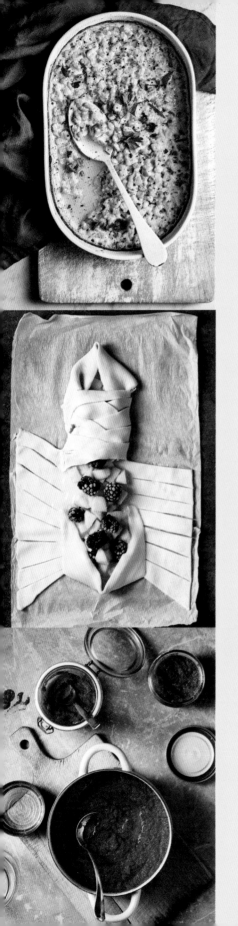

THE
RECIPES

POULTRY

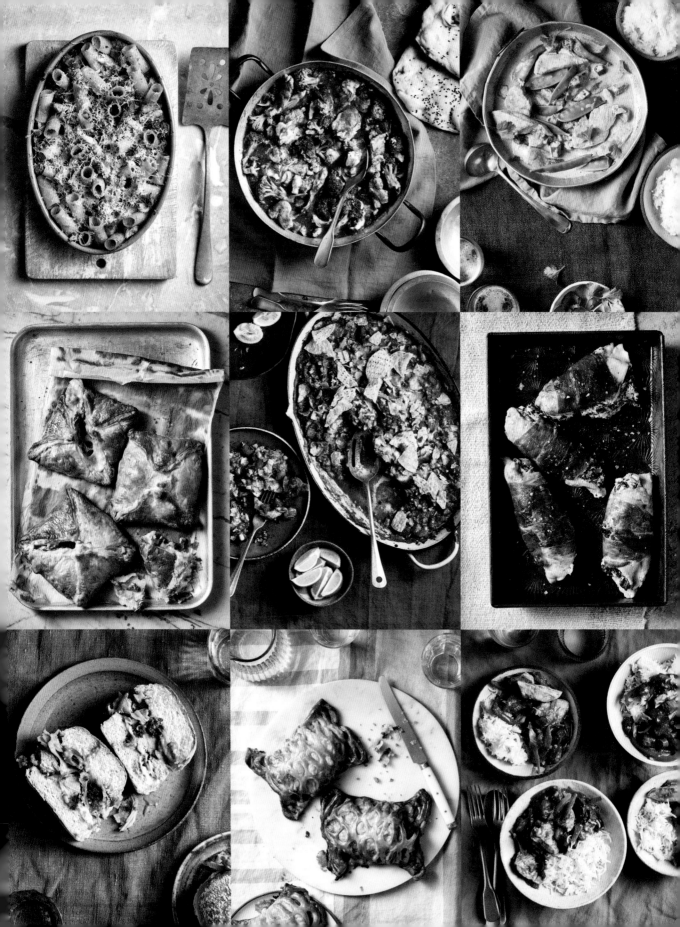

POULTRY

Versatile, quick to cook and liked by everyone, chicken is a mainstay ingredient of any busy family cook. In my house, it keeps even the fussiest of appetites happy and is the protein that I cook more than any other. In this chapter you will find lots of simple, delicious recipes for meals made with chicken that can be prepared ahead of time and pulled out of the freezer as needed.

As with all the recipes in this book, each meal is paired with another, so you can easily batch two dishes at once – making one for now and one for later. At the end of the chapter you'll find a plan for cooking ten delicious chicken recipes in one hour, making it possible to make two weeks' worth of delicious chicken-based dinners in just 60 minutes!

CHICKEN, ASPARAGUS & EMMENTAL PARCELS

P

PREP: 15 MINUTES
COOK: 25 MINUTES
SERVES 4

2 sheets ready-rolled puff
  pastry
1 x 295g can condensed
  cream of chicken soup
½ cup (50g) grated
  Emmental cheese
8 asparagus spears, cut into
  2.5cm (1in) pieces
1 cup (155g) frozen peas
1 egg, beaten, to cook

These delicious parcels are perfect for those days when you want the comfort of a pie, but don't have the time or energy to make one. They can be assembled quickly in advance and then cooked directly from frozen. If you're vegetarian or trying to cut down on meat, these are just as delicious made with mushroom soup instead of chicken.

If you are also making the Chicken Lattices, it is best to make the Chicken, Asparagus & Emmental Parcels first to avoid any cross contamination from the raw chicken.

01 Unroll the pastry sheets and cut each in half, leaving you with four roughly square pieces. If the pieces aren't quite square, trim the longer sides to even them up. Set aside.

02 Put the soup, Emmental cheese, asparagus and peas in a bowl and stir to combine. Now scoop a quarter of the mixture (about ½ cup) into the centre of each of the squares of pastry.

03 Bring up opposite corners of the squares of pastry and press them together to seal in the centre. Now work your way down the seams to seal the pastry and completely enclose the filling.

TO COOK: Transfer the parcels to a lined baking sheet and brush the tops with the egg wash. Cook in an oven preheated to 180°C/350°F/gas mark 4 for 20–25 minutes, until crisp and golden. Serve with vegetables of your choice alongside.

TO FREEZE: Carefully wrap each of the parcels in clingfilm, then transfer to a labelled plastic bag and freeze flat for up to 3 months.

TO COOK FROM FROZEN: These can be cooked from frozen. Place on a lined baking sheet and brush with beaten egg. Cook in an oven preheated to 180°C/350°F/gas mark 4 for 30–35 minutes, until golden. Serve with vegetables alongside.

CHICKEN, CHEESE & HAM PASTRY LATTICES

P

PREP: 20 MINUTES
COOK: 35 MINUTES
SERVES 4

1 sheet ready-rolled puff pastry
4 skinless, boneless chicken breasts
4 x 1cm- (½in-) thick slices cheddar cheese
4 slices ham
1 egg, beaten, to cook

Zhuzh it Up!
Substitute the ham for slices of prosciutto and change the cheese to slices of mozzarella for a more luxurious result.

This is one of those recipes that looks much harder than it actually is, all thanks to a bit of pastry wizardry! These are great to have stocked in the freezer, so I usually double the quantity and make eight lattices at once – it only takes a moment to make the extra ones as all the ingredients are already laid out.

01 Unroll the pastry sheet and cut into quarters, leaving you with four roughly square pieces. If the pieces aren't quite square, trim the longer sides to even up the pieces.

02 Using a lattice cutter, roll over the pieces of pastry, or alternatively use a sharp knife to cut 2cm (1in) slits in staggered rows 1cm (½in) apart. Gently pull the pastry apart so that the lattice shape opens up.

03 Line a baking tray with greaseproof paper and evenly space the chicken breasts on it. Place a slice of ham on each piece of chicken, then top each with a slice of cheddar cheese. Finally, top each stack with a piece of the latticed pastry, opening it up so that the top and sides of each chicken breast are enclosed.

TO SERVE: Brush the top of each pastry lattice with beaten egg, then transfer to an oven preheated to 200°C/400°F/gas mark 6 for 30–35 minutes, until golden, juicy and tender. Serve hot with vegetables of your choice alongside.

TO FREEZE: Transfer the uncooked lattices to a labelled freezer bag and freeze flat for up to 3 months.

TO COOK FROM FROZEN: Remove the chicken lattices from the freezer and allow to defrost completely, then brush with beaten egg and cook as described, left.

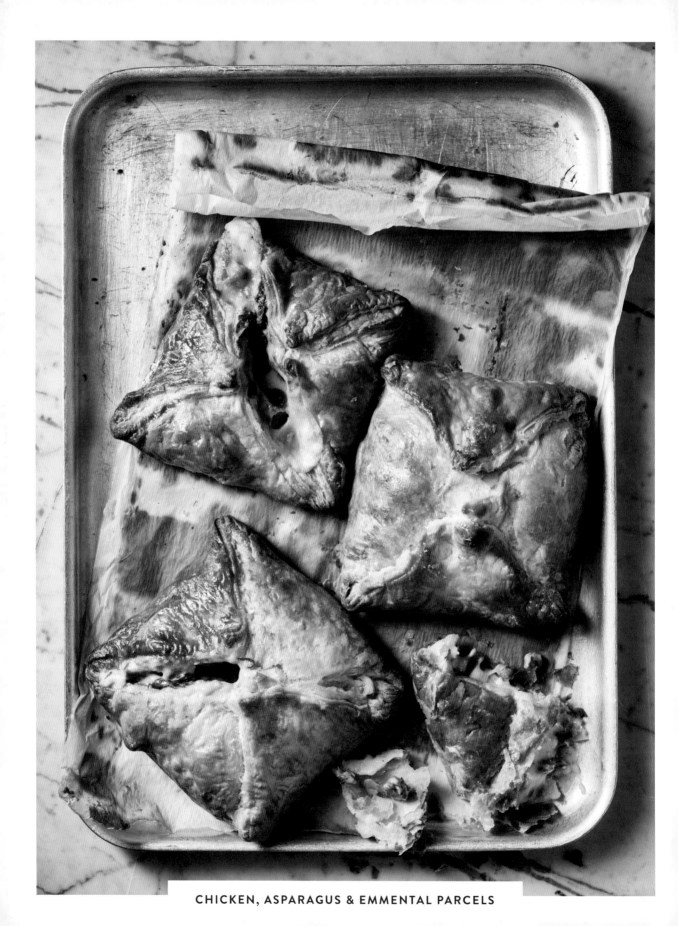

CHICKEN, ASPARAGUS & EMMENTAL PARCELS

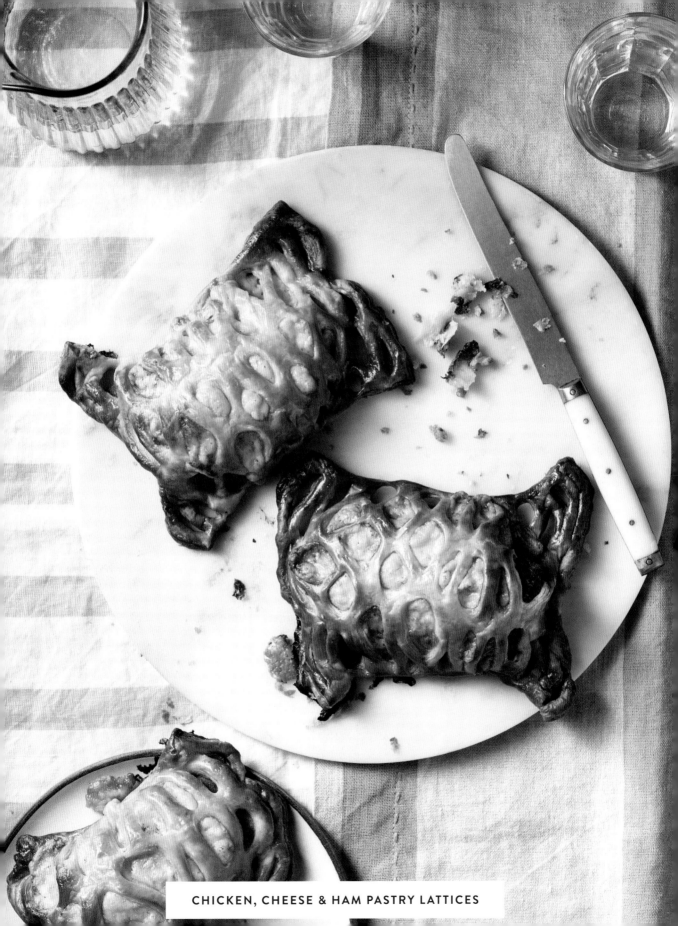

CHICKEN, CHEESE & HAM PASTRY LATTICES

CHICKEN, TOMATO & CHORIZO PASTA BAG

PREP: 10 MINUTES
COOK: 15 MINUTES
SERVES 4

splash of olive oil
1 cup (115g) chopped,
 frozen onions
2 skinless, boneless chicken
 breasts, cut into 5mm
 (¼in) slices
¼ cup (115g) bacon lardons
¼ cup (120g) frozen, diced
 chorizo
½ cup (120ml) Red Pesto
 (see page 221) or 100g
 store-bought, sundried
 tomato pesto
70g sundried tomatoes in
 oil, drained
3¾ cups (300g) penne
 pasta, to serve

Pull this bag out of the freezer in the morning and you can have a hearty evening meal on the table in the evening in the time it takes to cook a pan of pasta. Make this alongside the 'Nduja pasta bag (opposite) and you'll have two tasty, sustaining meals ready to go in next to no time.

01 Heat a splash of olive oil in a large pan over a medium-high heat, then add the onions and chicken and cook, stirring occasionally, until browned, about 5 minutes.

Clear away the chopping boards and knives from prepping the raw chicken and clean the kitchen worktops, then make this and the 'Nduja Pasta Bag alongside each other on the hob. The stages are very similar, so it is very easy to make both dishes at the same time.

02 Once the chicken has browned, add the bacon lardons and chorizo and stir through, then cook, stirring occasionally, until browned. Stir through the pesto and sundried tomatoes, then remove the pan from the heat.

TO COOK: If you are making this to serve now, simply cook the pasta in boiling water according to packet instructions, until tender. Stir the pasta through the chicken and pesto mixture, then divide between serving bowls and serve warm.

TO FREEZE: Set the chicken and pesto mixture aside until cooled to room temperature, then transfer to a labelled freezer bag and freeze flat for up to 3 months.

TO COOK FROM FROZEN: Remove the bag from the freezer and leave to completely defrost in the fridge. Once defrosted, transfer to a pan and cook until piping hot. Cook the pasta in a separate pan, then combine as described in the *To Cook* section, left.

'NDUJA PASTA BAG

PREP: 10 MINUTES
COOK: 15 MINUTES
SERVES 4

splash of olive oil
2 cups (230g) frozen,
  chopped onions
1 tsp frozen, chopped garlic
4–5 tbsp 'nduja spread
1½ cups (300g) cherry
  tomatoes, quartered
1 smoked sausage, sliced
4 cups (400g) rigatoni
  pasta, to serve
4 tbsp grated Parmesan
  cheese, to serve

'Nduja is a spicy paste made with pork and chilli from Calabria in Italy. You will find it beside the jars of pesto in the supermarket.

01 Heat a splash of olive oil in a large pan over a medium-high heat, then add the onions and garlic and cook, stirring occasionally, until softened, 3–4 minutes.

02 Add the 'nduja to the pan and stir until the onions are coated, then add the tomatoes and cook, stirring occasionally, for 5 minutes.

TO COOK: If you are making this to serve now, stir in the smoked sausage and keep warm while you cook the pasta. Stir the cooked pasta through the 'nduja and sausage mixture, then divide between serving bowls, scatter with Parmesan and serve warm.

TO FREEZE: Set the mixture aside until cooled to room temperature, then stir through the smoked sausage and transfer to a labelled freezer bag. Freeze flat for up to 3 months.

TO COOK FROM FROZEN: Remove the bag from the freezer and leave to completely defrost in the fridge. Once defrosted, transfer to a pan and cook until piping hot. Cook the pasta in a separate pan, then combine as described in the *To Cook* section, left.

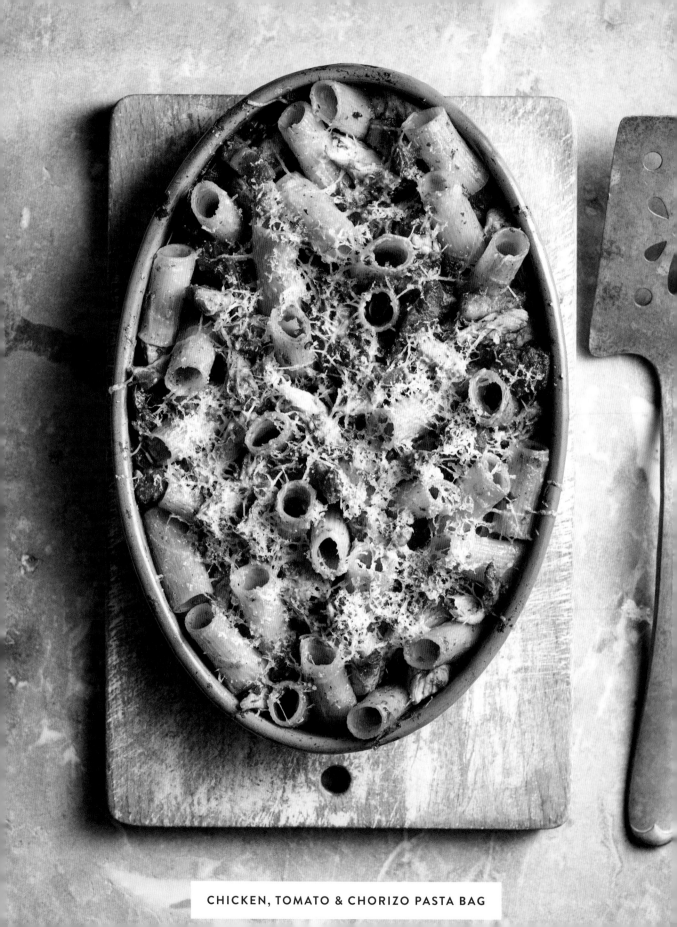

CHICKEN, TOMATO & CHORIZO PASTA BAG

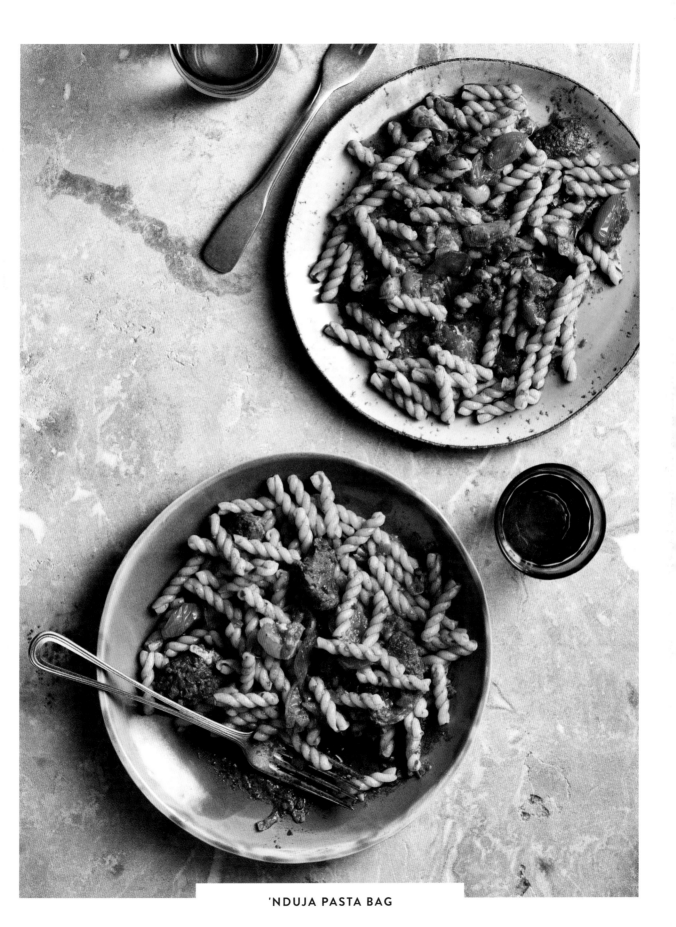

'NDUJA PASTA BAG

MEXICAN TRAYBAKE

PREP: 5 MINUTES
COOK: 25 MINUTES
SERVES 4

4 skinless, boneless chicken
  breasts, cut into 5mm
  (¼in) slices
1 x 30g pack taco or fajita
  seasoning
1 x 300g jar tomato salsa
2 cups (280g) frozen
  sweetcorn
1 x 400g can chopped
  tomatoes, drained
  through a sieve
1 cup (175g) frozen, sliced
  peppers (optional)
1 cup (90g) grated cheddar
  cheese
3 handfuls tortilla chips,
  crushed

This tasty recipe requires no cooking on the day that you assemble it for the freezer. It can then simply be defrosted and popped in the oven on the day that you want to serve it. What could be simpler?

TO COOK: Put the chicken in the base of a large baking dish, scatter over the taco or fajita seasoning and give the mixture a stir to coat the chicken in the spices. Add the salsa, sweetcorn, chopped tomatoes and peppers to the dish and stir again to combine. Scatter over the cheese, followed by the crushed tortilla chips. Bake in an oven preheated to 200°C/400°F/gas mark 6 for 25 minutes, until the chicken is cooked through and the cheese topping is golden and bubbling.

TO FREEZE: Put the chicken in a large, labelled freezer bag and scatter over the taco or fajita seasoning, rubbing the sides of the bag to coat the chicken in the spices. Add the salsa, sweetcorn, chopped tomatoes and peppers to the bag and give everything a shake to combine. Freeze flat for up to 3 months.

TO COOK FROM FROZEN: Remove the bag from the freezer and allow to defrost fully in the fridge. Once defrosted, tip the mixture into a large baking dish, scatter over the cheese and crushed tortillas and cook as described in the *To Cook* section, above.

CAJUN PORK STEAKS WITH PEPPERS

M

PREP: 5 MINUTES
COOK: 30 MINUTES
SERVES 4

2 tbsp plus 2 tsp smoky
  Cajun rub (available in the
  spice aisle)
2 tbsp olive oil
4 pork loin steaks
2 cups (350g) frozen,
  sliced peppers
1 x 400g can chopped
  tomatoes

This is such an easy recipe that I always double up and store two batches in the freezer for a no-fuss midweek meal. If you don't like pork steaks, simply substitute for chicken or beef. This is great served with Made-in-Advance Baked Potatoes (see page 193), some ready-made mash or a packet of microwavable Mexican rice.

01 Put 2 tbsp of the smoky Cajun rub in a bowl with the olive oil and combine to form a paste. Pour the oil and spice paste over the pork steaks and use your hands to ensure they are well coated. Set aside.

02 In the same bowl that the spice paste was made in, combine the remaining smoky Cajun rub and the chopped tomatoes.

TO COOK: Lay the spice-coated pork steaks in a large baking dish and top with the sliced peppers, then pour over the spiced tomato mixture. Transfer to an oven preheated to 180°C/350°F/gas mark 4 and cook for 25–30 minutes, until the pork is tender. Serve hot.

TO FREEZE: Put the spice-coated pork steaks in a large, labelled freezer bag, followed by the peppers and spiced tomato mixture. Give the bag a shake to combine the flavours, then freeze flat for up to 3 months.

TO COOK FROM FROZEN: Remove the bag from the freezer and allow to defrost in the fridge. Once defrosted, tip the mixture into a baking dish and cook as described in the *To Cook* section, left.

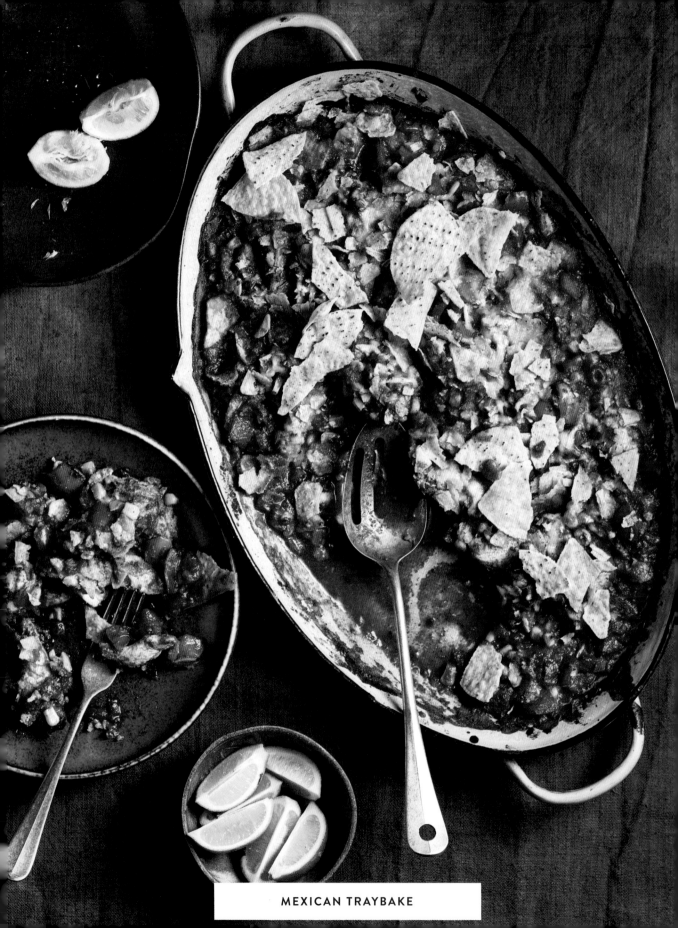

MEXICAN TRAYBAKE

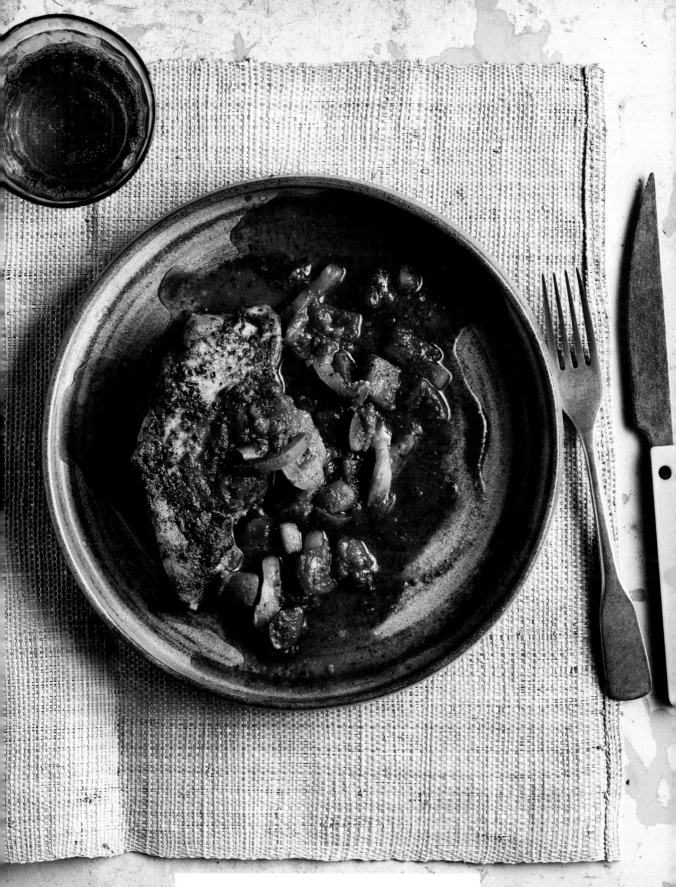

CAJUN PORK STEAKS WITH PEPPERS

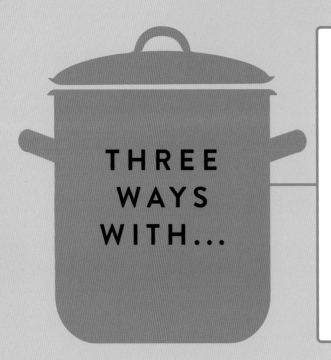

THREE WAYS WITH...

CAJUN PORK STEAKS

Now that you've prepared your Cajun Pork Steaks, what are you going to do with them? Below are three simple ideas for different ways of serving them that will keep mealtimes feeling fresh and different every time!

CAJUN PORK STEAKS WITH MASHED POTATOES

1 x quantity Cajun Pork Steaks with Peppers (p.47)
1 x 400g pack ready-made mashed potatoes
2 cups (300g) frozen, mixed vegetables, to serve

01 Prepare the pork steaks as described on page 47.
02 When the pork steaks have almost finished cooking, heat the mashed potato and frozen, mixed vegetables in the microwave according to packet instructions.
03 Serve the pork steaks with the mashed potatoes and cooked veg alongside.

CAJUN PORK PANINIS WITH CORN ON THE COB

1 x quantity Cajun Pork Steaks
   with Peppers (p.47)
4 panini rolls, sliced open
4 corn on the cob
2–3 large tomatoes, sliced
sliced gherkins, to taste
   (optional)

01 Prepare the pork steaks as described on page 47.

02 When the pork steaks have almost finished cooking, put the corn in a pan of boiling water and cook for 5–10 minutes, until tender.

03 Slice the cooked pork into bite-sized pieces and spoon into the panini rolls, then top with a few of the cooked peppers, a couple of slices of tomato and some gherkins, if using. Serve hot with the corn on the cob on the side.

CAJUN PORK STEAKS WITH NOODLES

1 x quantity Cajun Pork Steaks
   with Peppers (p.47)
2–3 nests dried noodles
mixed salad leaves, to serve
your choice of salad dressing

01 Prepare the pork steaks as described on page 47.

02 When the pork steaks have almost finished cooking, cook the noodles in boiling water according to packet instructions.

03 Drain the cooked noodles and divide between four serving bowls, then top each with a Cajun pork steak and a spoonful of cooked peppers, plus any juices from the pan. Serve hot with a bowl of dressed salad leaves alongside.

THAI GREEN CHICKEN CURRY

PREP: 5 MINUTES
COOK: 15 MINUTES
SERVES 4

splash of sesame or vegetable oil
3 skinless, boneless chicken breasts
about 6 tbsp Thai green curry paste (check label for guidelines, as different brands vary in strength)
1 cup (100g) frozen, chopped okra
1 x 400g can coconut milk
1 cup (100g) mangetout
cooked rice or noodles, to serve
1 small bunch coriander, chopped, to serve

Ready-made curry pastes are a great way of adding an instant punch of flavour to a dish and are far quicker than making your own pastes from scratch. The two Thai curries on the following pages are wonderfully fragrant and very quick to make.

If you are also making the Thai Red Curry, put the sweet potatoes on to boil first, then continue with the Green Curry.

01 Place the chicken breasts on a board and slice, on the diagonal, into 1cm (½in) slices. Heat a splash of sesame or vegetable oil in a frying pan, then add the sliced chicken and cook, stirring, for 3–4 minutes, until sealed.

If you are also making the Thai Red Curry, drain the sweet potatoes now, then set another pan on the stove and make the sauces for both curries side by side.

02 If you are making the curry to eat straight away, cook the rice or noodles according to packet instructions now. Add the curry paste and okra to the pan with the chicken and stir until everything is coated in the paste. Pour in the coconut milk, then add the mangetout, stir to combine, and leave to simmer for 5–10 minutes, until the chicken and vegetables are tender.

TO SERVE: The curry is now ready to be served, spooned over a bed of cooked rice or noodles and garnished with freshly chopped coriander.

TO FREEZE: Set the curry aside to cool to room temperature, then spoon into a labelled freezer bag and freeze flat for up to 3 months.

TO COOK FROM FROZEN: Remove the freezer bag of curry from the freezer and allow to defrost fully in the fridge. The defrosted curry can be reheated in a pan on the stove until piping hot, then served as described in the *To Serve* section, left.

THAI RED SWEET POTATO CURRY

PREP: 5 MINUTES
COOK: 20 MINUTES
SERVES 4

1 x 500g bag frozen,
  chopped sweet potatoes
splash of sesame or
  vegetable oil
1 cup (115g) frozen,
  chopped onions
about 6 tbsp Thai red curry
  paste (check label for
  guidelines, as different
  brands vary in strength)
1 red pepper, sliced
1 cup (100g) green beans
1 x 400g can coconut milk
cooked rice or noodles,
  to serve
1 small bunch coriander,
  chopped, to serve

01 Bring a large pan of water to the boil, then add the sweet potato and leave to cook for 10–12 minutes, until just tender.

02 Heat a splash of sesame or vegetable oil in a deep frying pan or wok, then add the onions and cook, stirring, for 4–5 minutes, until golden. Add the curry paste, red pepper and green beans and stir until the vegetables are well coated in the paste.

03 Drain the sweet potato through a colander and add to the frying pan or wok along with the coconut milk. Stir the mixture to combine, then leave to simmer for 5–10 minutes, until the vegetables are tender.

Note
For a milder, child-friendly version of this curry, simply stir some creme fraiche through the sauce before serving.

TO SERVE: The curry is now ready to be served, spooned over a bed of cooked rice or noodles and garnished with freshly chopped coriander.

TO FREEZE: Set the curry aside to cool to room temperature, then spoon into a labelled freezer bag and freeze flat for up to 3 months.

TO COOK FROM FROZEN: Remove the freezer bag of curry from the freezer and allow to defrost fully in the fridge. The defrosted curry can be reheated in a pan on the stove until piping hot, then served as described in the *To Serve* section, left.

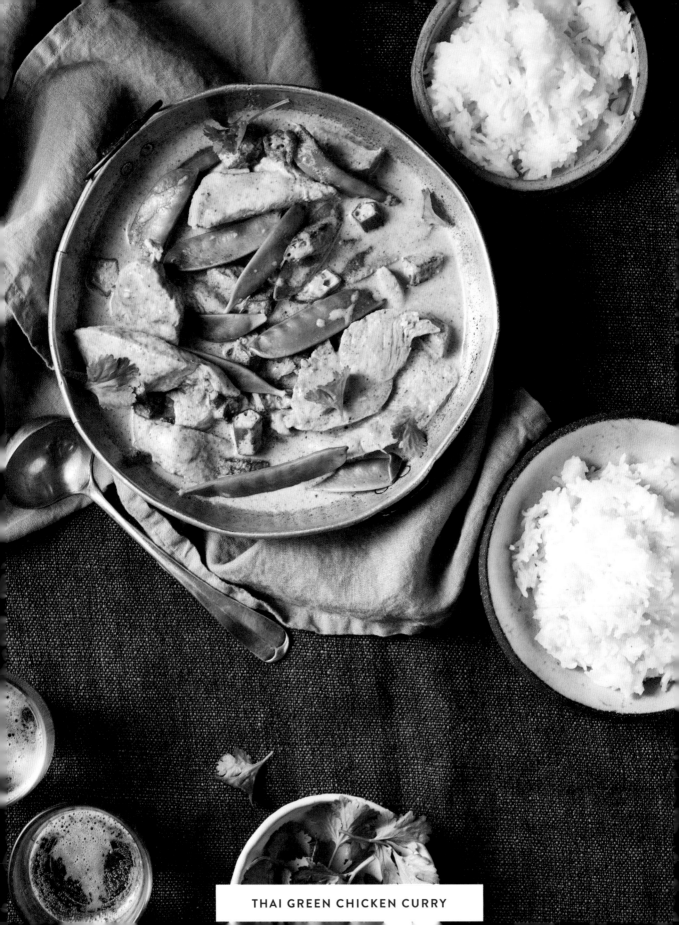

THAI GREEN CHICKEN CURRY

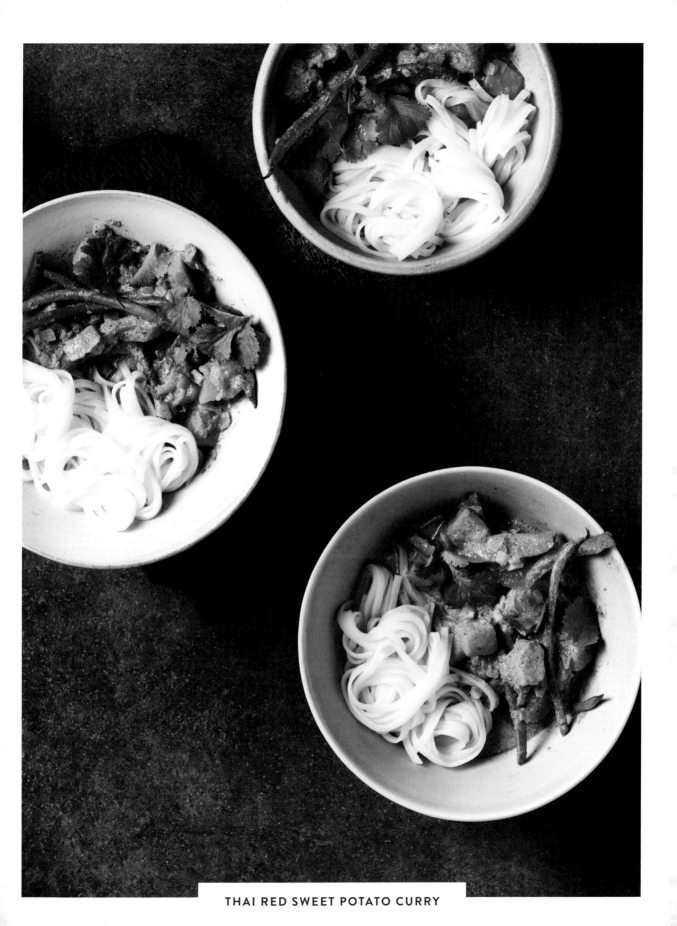

THAI RED SWEET POTATO CURRY

CHICKEN & BROCCOLI TIKKA MASALA

PREP: 5 MINUTES
COOK: 15 MINUTES
SERVES 4

splash of vegetable oil
2 cups (230g) frozen,
    chopped onions
3 skinless, boneless chicken
    or turkey breasts, cut into
    bite-sized pieces
1 x 400g can chopped
    tomatoes
1 head broccoli, cut into
    small florets
½ jar (150g) tikka masala
    spice paste (check label
    for guidelines, as different
    brands vary in strength)
To Serve:
1 cup (200g) of crème
    fraiche (optional)
cooked rice
naan breads

When cooking for children you often have to limit the spice to cater for their tastes, but with these recipes you can make two curries side-by-side, one spicy and one mild, meaning that everyone is happy!

I make these two curries at the same time — simply place the 2 piles of ingredients out on the side, set two pans on the stove and work through the steps side-by-side.

01 Heat a splash of vegetable oil in a deep frying pan or wok over a medium heat, then add the onions and cook for 2–3 minutes, until softened. Add the chicken or turkey and cook, stirring occasionally, until sealed.

02 Add the chopped tomatoes, broccoli and tikka masala paste along with ½ cup (120ml) of water and stir to combine. Bring to a gentle simmer, then leave to cook for 10 minutes, stirring occasionally, until the meat is cooked through.

TO SERVE: If you want a creamier tasting curry, stir through the crème fraiche, then serve with cooked rice and naan breads alongside.

TO FREEZE: Set the curry aside to cool to room temperature, then spoon into a large, labelled freezer bag, seal and freeze flat for up to 3 months. I freeze naan breads alongside, so both can be defrosted at the same time.

TO COOK FROM FROZEN: Remove the curry from the freezer and leave to defrost fully in the fridge, then reheat in a pan on the stove for 15–20 minutes, until piping hot. Serve as described in the *To Serve* section, left.

CHICKEN, OKRA & PEPPER JALFREZI

PREP: 5 MINUTES
COOK: 10 MINUTES
SERVES 4

splash of vegetable oil
2 cups (230g) frozen,
 sliced red onions
1 tsp frozen, chopped garlic
1 tsp frozen, chopped
 chillies
3 skinless, boneless chicken
 or turkey breasts, cut into
 bite-sized pieces
1 x 400g can chopped
 tomatoes
1½ cups (150g) frozen,
 chopped okra
1 cup (175g) frozen, sliced
 peppers
½ jar (150g) jalfrezi spice
 paste (check label for
 guidelines, as different
 brands vary in strength)

I make these two curries at the same time — simply place the 2 piles of ingredients out on the side, set two pans on the stove and work through the steps side by side.

01 Heat a splash of vegetable oil in a deep frying pan or wok over a medium heat, then add the onions, garlic and chillies and cook for 2–3 minutes, until softened. Add the chicken or turkey and cook, stirring occasionally, until sealed.

02 Add the chopped tomatoes, okra, sliced peppers and jalfrezi spice paste along with ½ cup (120ml) of water and stir to combine, Bring to a gentle simmer, then leave to cook for 10 minutes, stirring occasionally.

Zhuzh it Up!
Stir through a few generous spoonfuls of crème fraiche to temper the heat and make this a dish the whole family will enjoy.

TO SERVE: The curry is now ready to serve with cooked rice and naan breads alongside.

TO FREEZE: Set the curry aside to cool to room temperature, then spoon into a large, labelled freezer bag, seal and freeze flat for up to 3 months. I freeze naan breads alongside, so both can be defrosted at the same time.

TO COOK FROM FROZEN: Remove the curry from the freezer and leave to defrost fully in the fridge, then reheat in a pan on the stove for 15–20 minutes, until piping hot. Serve as described in the *To Serve* section, left.

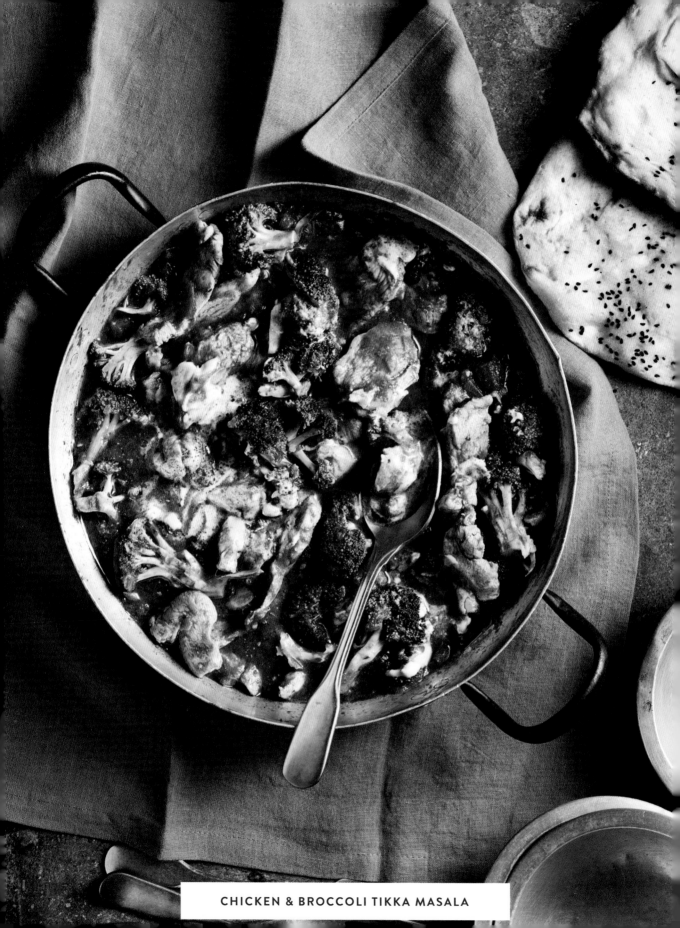

CHICKEN & BROCCOLI TIKKA MASALA

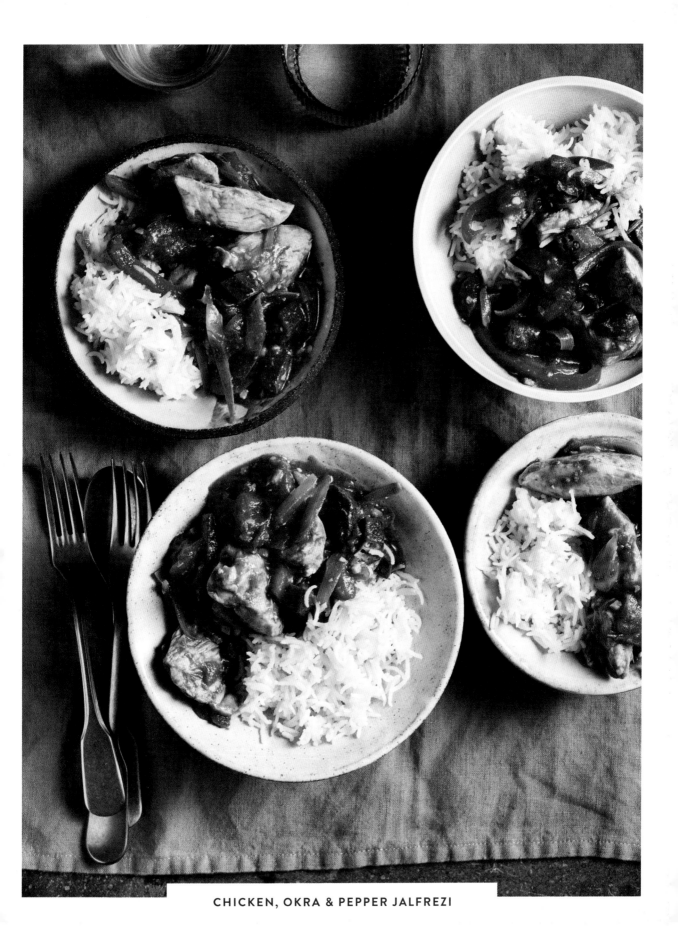

CHICKEN, OKRA & PEPPER JALFREZI

10 CHICKEN MEALS IN 1 HOUR

Are you ready to cook ten chicken-based family meals in just 60 minutes? You will be making five recipes, each of which is doubled up to feed eight people, so just has to be split into two meals before freezing. The recipes are a mixture of cooked and no-cook meals, so while one recipe is bubbling away on the stove or cooking in the oven, you can be prepping the next for the freezer.

The shopping list on the opposite page includes everything you need and I've scaled up the ingredients so you know what size pack of each ingredient to buy. Once you have your shopping, lay the ingredients out in piles according to the groupings overleaf, so that you have exactly what you need for each recipe to hand. Then, simply follow the numbered guide and you can't go wrong!

Don't panic if this takes you more than an hour the first time you cook it – you will get quicker each time you make it. So, roll up your sleeves, get cooking and think about the time you'll be saving yourself in the future!

YOU WILL BE MAKING:

BRIDE'S CHICKEN
CHICKEN BALTI
CHICKEN ENCHILADAS
MOZZARELLA HASSELBACK CHICKEN
HUNTER'S CHICKEN

SHOPPING LIST

Fresh

5 tomatoes

3 heads broccoli

2 x 300g packs button mushrooms

1 lemon

small bunch fresh basil

34 skinless, boneless chicken breasts

8 rashers of smoked back bacon

1 x 500g pack grated cheddar cheese

2 mozzarella balls

Frozen

1 x 500g pack frozen, sliced peppers

1 x 500g pack frozen, chopped onions

1 x 900g pack frozen, chopped spinach

Storecupboard

5 x 400g tins chopped tomatoes

4 x 295g tins condensed soup
 (cream of mushroom or chicken)

8 corn tortilla wraps

1 bottle olive or vegetable oil

1 jar mayonnaise

1 x bottle BBQ sauce

1 jar tomato salsa

1 x 280g jar balti paste

1 packet fajita/taco seasoning

1 jar medium curry powder

INGREDIENTS

GET ORGANIZED! Before you start make sure that your kitchen surfaces are cleared down, then lay all the ingredients out in individual piles according to the groupings on these two pages.

BRIDE'S CHICKEN

6 skinless, boneless chicken breasts

2 heads broccoli, cut into small florets

4 x 295g cans condensed cream of mushroom or chicken soup

4 tsp lemon juice

4 tsp medium curry powder

6 cups (360g) button mushrooms

2 cups (480ml) mayonnaise

CHICKEN BALTI & CHICKEN ENCHILADAS

For both dishes:

5 tbsp olive or vegetable oil

4 cups (460g) frozen, chopped onions

12 skinless, boneless chicken breasts, cut into bite-sized pieces

For the Balti:

24 cubes frozen, chopped spinach

4 x 400g cans chopped tomatoes

1 x 280g jar balti spice paste

1 head broccoli, cut into florets (optional)

For the Enchiladas:

1 x 30g pack fajita/taco seasoning

8 corn tortilla wraps

2 cups (180g) grated cheddar cheese

1 x 400g can chopped tomatoes

1 cup (240ml) store-bought Mexican salsa

2 cups (150g) sliced frozen peppers (optional)

HUNTER'S CHICKEN

2 cups (180g) grated cheddar cheese

2 cups (480ml) store-bought BBQ sauce

8 skinless, boneless chicken breasts

8 rashers smoked back bacon

MOZZARELLA HASSELBACK CHICKEN

8 skinless, boneless chicken breasts

2 balls mozzarella, sliced

5 tomatoes, sliced

1 small bunch basil, leaves picked

METHOD

BRIDE'S CHICKEN

01 Lay a large sheet of foil on the work surface and place six chicken breasts onto it. Fold the foil over and scrunch the edges to form a sealed parcel, then transfer to an oven preheated to 180°C/350°F/gas mark 4 for 35–40 minutes, until the chicken is cooked.

CHICKEN BALTI & CHICKEN ENCHILADAS

02 Heat the oil in a large pan over a medium heat, then add the frozen onions and cook, stirring, for 2–3 minutes, until softened. Add the chopped chicken to the pan and cook, stirring occasionally, for 10 minutes, until sealed.

HUNTER'S CHICKEN

03 While the chicken above is cooking, assemble the Hunter's Chicken. Divide the grated cheese between two small freezer bags and seal, then divide the BBQ sauce between another two freezer bags and seal.

04 Wrap each of the 8 chicken breasts with a rasher of bacon. Place two large sheets of foil on the counter and place four wrapped chicken breasts on each. Fold over each sheet of foil and crimp the edges together to form two parcels, then place each parcel in a large, labelled freezer bag along with one bag of the cheese and one bag of the BBQ sauce. Seal and freeze flat for up to 3 months.

MOZZARELLA HASSELBACK CHICKEN

05 To assemble the Mozzarella Hasselback chicken, set the chicken breasts on a chopping board, then cut horizontal slices three quarters of the way through the chicken at 1cm (½in) intervals along the breasts.

06 Insert slices of mozzarella and tomato alternately into each of the cuts, then slot a few basil leaves along each breast. Place two large sheets of foil on the counter and place four filled chicken breasts on each. Fold over each sheet of foil and crimp the edges together to form two parcels, then place each parcel in a large, labelled freezer bag. Freeze flat for up to 3 months.

BRIDE'S CHICKEN CONTINUED ...

07 The chicken in the oven should now be cooked. Remove and set aside on the counter to cool slightly while you complete the Balti and Enchilada recipes.

BALTI & ENCHILADAS CONTINUED ...

08 The chicken and onion in the pan should now be cooked. Transfer half to a large bowl and set aside to make the Chicken Enchiladas.

09 Return the remaining chicken and onion mixture to the heat and add the spinach cubes, chopped tomatoes, balti paste, broccoli, if using, and scant 1 cup (200ml) of water. Leave to cook, stirring occasionally, until the spinach has thawed and the mixture is bubbling. Set the Balti aside to cool.

10 Add the fajita seasoning to the remaining chicken mixture and stir to combine. Heat the tortilla wraps in the microwave for 15 seconds, then divide the spiced chicken mixture between the wraps. Scatter over half of the grated cheese, then roll the tortillas around the filling and arrange, seam-side down, in two large baking dishes or foil trays.

11 Combine the chopped tomatoes and salsa in a bowl, then pour over the Enchiladas. Top with the sliced peppers, if using, and scatter over the remaining cheese. Set aside to cool to room temperature while you complete the Bride's Chicken.

BRIDE'S CHICKEN CONTINUED ...

12 Add the broccoli florets to a pan of boiling water, then leave to cook for 2 minutes.

13 Shred the cooked chicken breasts into a large bowl, then add the cooked broccoli, condensed soup, lemon juice, curry powder, button mushrooms and mayonnaise, then give everything a good stir to combine.

14 Divide the mixture between two large, labelled freezer bags, seal and freeze flat for up to 3 months.

BALTI & ENCHILADAS CONTINUED ...

15 Once cooled, divide the Balti mixture between two large, labelled freezer bags, seal and freeze flat for up to 3 months.

16 Once the Enchiladas have cooled, wrap in a layer of clingfilm followed by a layer of foil, then label and freeze flat for up to 3 months.

Congratulations!
You now have 10 evening meals
ready for the freezer!

WHEN YOU COME TO COOK

Once cooked and frozen, all of these meals are best fully defrosted before cooking. All reheated meals should reach a temperature of 74°C/165°F. Always make sure any reheated food is piping hot before serving. Cooking times for each dish are listed below.

BRIDE'S CHICKEN

Once defrosted, transfer to a microwave-proof bowl and cook in the microwave on high for 4 minutes, until piping hot. Alternatively, transfer to a pan and heat over a medium-high heat for around 15 minutes, stirring occasionally, until piping hot.

CHICKEN BALTI

Once defrosted, transfer to a heatproof bowl and cook in the microwave on high for 4 minutes, until piping hot. Alternatively, transfer to a pan and heat over a medium-high heat for around 15 minutes, stirring occasionally, until piping hot.

ENCHILADAS

Once defrosted, transfer to an oven preheated to 180°C/350°F/gas mark 4 for 20–25 minutes, until piping hot.

HUNTER'S CHICKEN

Once defrosted, transfer the foil parcels to an oven preheated to 180°C/350°F/gas mark 4 for 20 minutes, then open the parcels, add the barbecue sauce and grated cheese and return to the oven for another 15 minutes until golden and bubbling.

MOZZARELLA HASSELBACK CHICKEN

Once defrosted, transfer the foil parcels to an oven preheated to 180°C/350°F/gas mark 4 for 30–35 minutes, until piping hot.

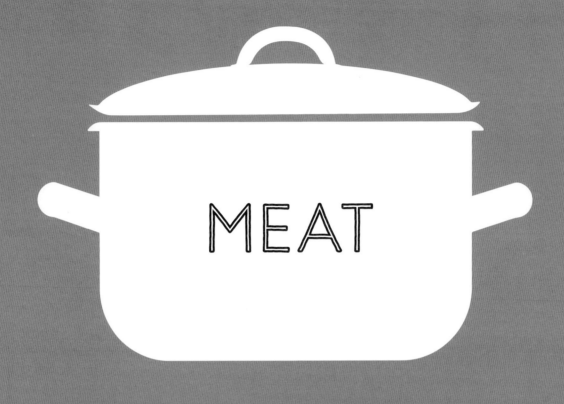

MEAT

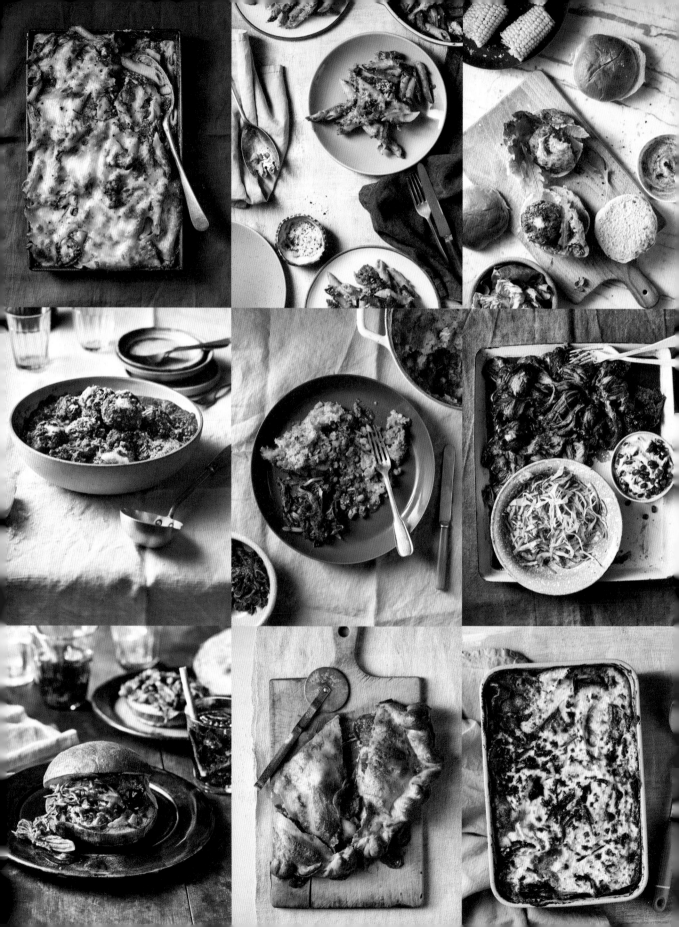

MEAT

From breakfast to dinner, there is something in this chapter for every time of the day. I love the two breakfast dishes at the start of this chapter as they clearly demonstrate the full benefits of batching in advance. Making a full cooked breakfast when you have a houseful of people can be messy and longwinded, but preparing my Breakfast Quiche (p.71) or American Breakfast Hash (p.70) ahead of time, then defrosting in the fridge overnight when you have guests, means having an impressive breakfast on the table can be the work of moments.

This section contains some real batching classics – making meals such as chilli, cottage pie and lasagne is where most batchers cut their teeth, as they are all easy to make and freeze perfectly. I first started cooking multiple recipes at the same time after making many of the meals in this chapter over and over again, as I realized that they were made using similar ingredients. My method for ten mince meals in one hour, found at the end of this chapter, is definitely one of my most popular and works for any depth of pocket, whether you are on a tight budget or like to buy grass-fed organic beef from the butcher.

Don't be surprised if you find a sneaky dessert option or two in this chapter – sometimes something sweet twins well with a savoury recipe, such as with my savoury and sweet Calzones, so it makes sense to prepare them at the same time.

AMERICAN BREAKFAST HASH

PREP: 15 MINS
COOK: 45 MINS
SERVES 4–6

8 pork sausages
8 rashers of bacon
4 slices black pudding
2 cups (200g) frozen,
   cubed potatoes
12 white mushrooms,
   roughly chopped
12 cherry tomatoes
1 cup (175g) frozen, sliced
   peppers
To Serve:
4 eggs, beaten
splash of milk
2¼ cups (200g) grated
   cheddar cheese

I serve this for breakfast every year on Boxing Day, as it is perfect for pulling out of the freezer when you have a houseful of ravenous, bleary-eyed guests and need to get something delicious on the table in a hurry.

01 Preheat the oven to 200°C/400°F/gas mark 6 and line four baking sheets with foil.

02 Place the sausages, bacon, black pudding and frozen, cubed potatoes on separate baking trays, then transfer to the oven for 15–20 minutes, until cooked through. The ingredients will cook at different times, so you will need to keep an eye on each component and remove from the oven when it is ready.

If you are also making the Breakfast Quiche, cook the sausages, bacon and black pudding at the same time as those for the Hash.

03 Once all the components are cooked, set aside to cool then cut everything into bite-sized pieces.

TO COOK: Transfer the cooked ingredients, mushrooms, tomatoes and peppers to a roasting pan, cover with foil and cook at 200°C/400°F/gas 6 for 20 minutes. When the Hash is almost cooked, mix the eggs and milk and scramble over a low heat, then stir through the hash and scatter with cheese. Return to the oven, uncovered, for 5 minutes, until bubbling. Serve.

TO FREEZE: If you are making the dish ahead of time to store in the freezer, leave all of the cooked ingredients to cool, then place in a large, clearly labelled freezer bag along with the tomatoes, mushrooms and frozen peppers. Seal the bag flat and transfer to the freezer for up to 3 months.

TO COOK FROM FROZEN: Remove the Hash from the freezer and allow to completely defrost, then cook as described in the *To Cook* section, left.

BREAKFAST QUICHE

M

PREP: 15 MINS
COOK: 1 HR 15 MINS
SERVES 6–8

butter, for greasing
2 pork sausages
2 rashers of bacon
2 slices black pudding
1 x 500g block ready-
   made puff pastry
1½ cups (125g) pre-grated
   cheddar cheese
4 white mushrooms,
   roughly chopped
6 cherry tomatoes, roughly
   chopped
6 eggs, beaten
splash of milk
salt and freshly ground
   pepper, to taste

01 Preheat the oven to 180°C/350°F/gas mark 4, line a baking tray with foil and grease a 28cm (11in) diameter quiche tin with butter.

02 Place the sausages, bacon and black pudding on the prepared baking tray, transfer to the oven for 15–20 minutes, removing each component from the oven when it is ready. Do not turn off the oven.

03 Once all the components are cooked through, set aside to cool slightly then cut everything into bite-sized pieces.

04 On a lightly floured surface, roll out the pastry to a thickness of 5mm (¼in) and use to line the prepared quiche tin. Trim the pastry, ensuring that you leave a slight overhang as it will shrink during cooking. Prick all over with a fork.

05 Put half of the cheese in the base of the pastry-lined tin, then add the cooked meats followed by the chopped mushrooms and tomatoes.

06 Whisk the eggs with a splash of milk and season generously with salt and pepper, then pour the mixture into the tart tin. Scatter over the remaining cheese and transfer to the oven to cook. After 20 minutes, remove the Quiche from the oven and cover with foil, then return to the oven and cook for 35 minutes more, until the top is golden and well risen. Check that the Quiche is cooked through by pressing a fork into its centre, returning it to the oven for another 10 minutes if it is not fully set.

TO SERVE: Set the Quiche aside for 10 minutes to firm up, then slice and serve warm. Alternatively, set aside until cool and serve.

TO FREEZE: Leave to cool to room temperature, then wrap in clingfilm, label clearly and freeze flat for up to 1 month. Alternatively, freeze individual portions by slicing the Quiche and carefully wrapping each slice in clingfilm before freezing.

TO COOK FROM FROZEN: If whole, the Quiche can be reheated from frozen. Simply cover with foil and cook in a 180°C/400°F/gas mark 6 oven for 50 minutes, until piping hot all the way through. Individual slices should be left to defrost, then reheated in the oven until piping hot.

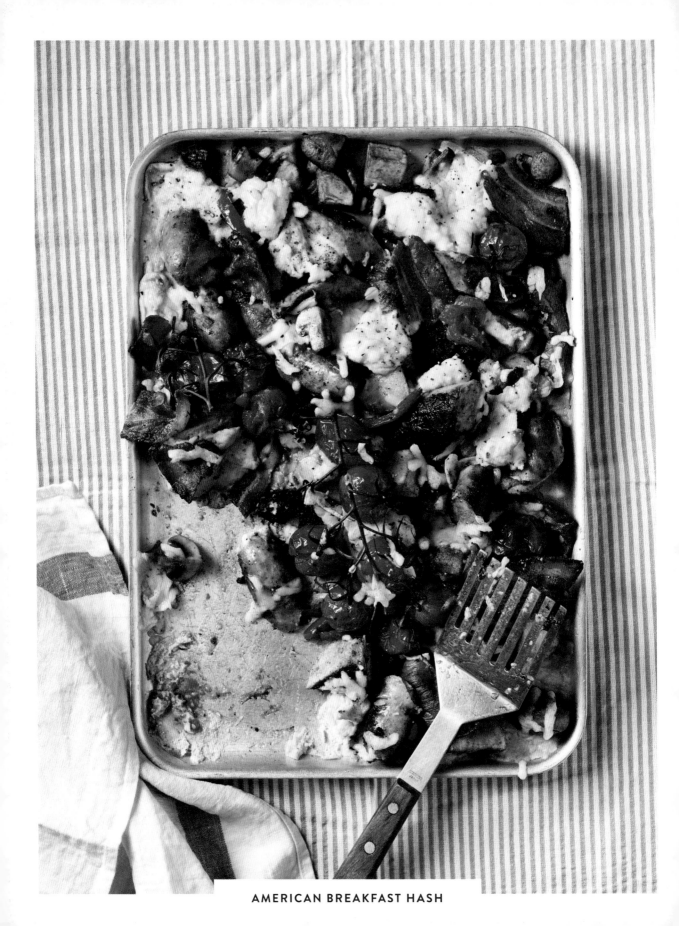

AMERICAN BREAKFAST HASH

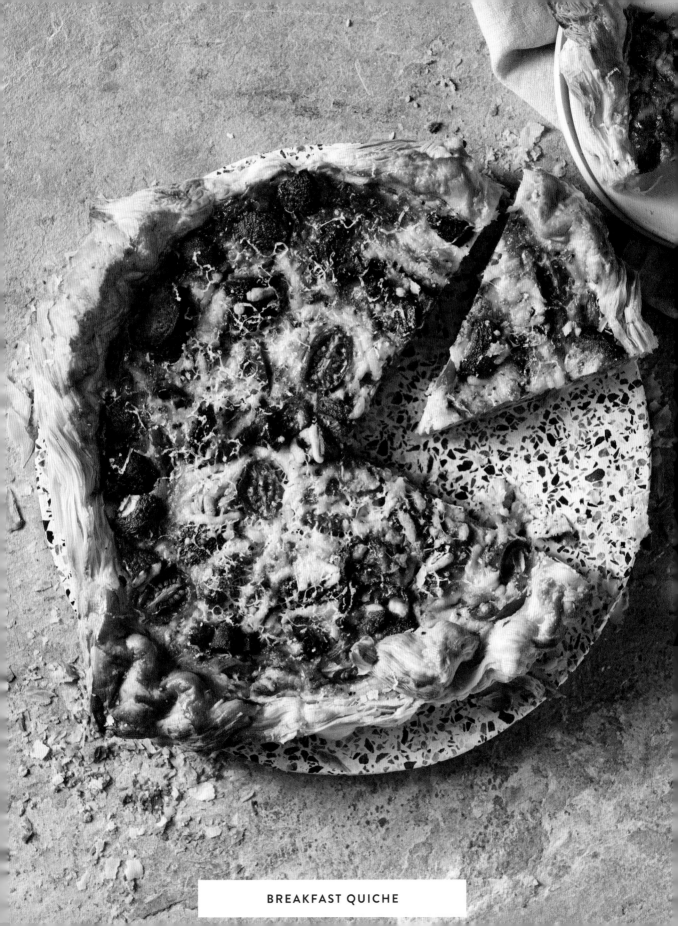

BREAKFAST QUICHE

FARMER'S WIFE'S SAVOURY PLAIT

PREP: 20 MINUTES
COOK: 40 MINUTES
SERVES 4–6

1 sheet fresh, ready-rolled
  puff pastry
190g (about ½ pack)
  sausage meat
3 tbsp store-bought
  caramelized onion
  chutney
1 apple, cored, halved and
  cut into slices (optional)
1 egg, beaten

This recipe was given to me by a local farmer's wife and it makes the perfect grab-and-go lunch or dinner on those hectic days when everyone seems to be going in different directions and just passing through the kitchen before heading off to another activity.

01 Unroll the sheet of puff pastry and set on the countertop, keeping it on its greaseproof lining paper.

02 Place the sausage meat in a long strip running lengthways down the middle third of the pastry, leaving a 2cm (¾in) gap at both ends.

03 Flatten the meat down slightly, then spoon the chutney along the sausage meat and lay the apple slices over the top, if using.

04 Using the picture on page 77 as a guide, use a sharp knife to make diagonal cuts every 2cm (¾in) along the length of the pastry on both sides of the filling.

05 Bring up the ends of the pastry and use them to secure the filling at the top and bottom, again using the image on page 77 as a guide.

06 Brush the edges of the pastry with the beaten egg, then start bringing the pastry strands into the centre, alternating sides so that the pieces overlap at the top and create a plait effect.

TO COOK: Slide the Plait, still on its greaseproof paper, onto a baking tray and brush the top and sides with beaten egg. Transfer to an oven preheated to 180°C/350°F/gas mark 4 and bake for 40 minutes, covering the top with foil if the pastry starts to catch. The Plait is now ready to slice and serve.

TO FREEZE: Bring up the sides of the greaseproof paper to encase the Plait, then wrap in clingfilm. You can label the clingfilm or transfer the Plait to a large, labelled freezer bag and freeze flat for up to 1 month.

TO COOK FROM FROZEN: This can be cooked from frozen. Unwrap the Plait and place on a lined baking tray, then brush the top and sides with beaten egg. Transfer to an oven preheated to 180°C/350°F/gas mark 4 and bake for 1 hour, covering the top with foil if the pastry starts to catch. The Plait is now ready to slice and serve.

APPLE & BLACKBERRY PLAIT

PREP: 20 MINUTES
COOK: 40 MINUTES
SERVES 4-6

1 sheet fresh, ready-rolled puff pastry
1 x 400g can apple pie filling (omit this if you are making the fresh filling)
1 cup (160g) frozen blackberries
1 egg, beaten
1 tsp caster sugar, to cook

If making your own apple filling:
2 bramley apples, peeled, cored and chopped into 2cm (¾in) cubes
2 tbsp caster sugar

This sweet plait is easy to make alongside the savoury version, as once you've got the hang of the technique you'll be able to knock these up really quickly! This is delicious served with a generous helping of ice cream or custard alongside.

01 If you are making your own filling, put the chopped apple and sugar in a small pan over a low heat and leave to cook, stirring occasionally, for around 10 minutes, until the apple is softened but still holding its shape.

02 Unroll the sheet of puff pastry and set on the countertop, keeping it on its greaseproof lining paper.

03 Place the fresh or canned apple filling in a long strip running lengthways down the middle third of the pastry, leaving a 2cm (¾in) gap at both ends. Dot the frozen blackberries along the length of the apple filling.

04 Using the picture on page 77 as a guide, use a sharp knife to make diagonal cuts every 2cm (¾in) along the length of the pastry on both sides of the filling.

05 Bring up the ends of the pastry and use them to secure the filling at the top and bottom.

06 Brush the edges of the pastry with the beaten egg, then start bringing the pastry strands into the centre, alternating sides so that the pieces overlap at the top and create a plait effect.

TO COOK: Slide the Plait, still on its greaseproof paper, onto a baking tray and brush the top and sides with beaten egg, then sprinkle over the caster sugar. Transfer to an oven preheated to 180°C/350°F/gas mark 4 and bake for 40 minutes, covering with foil if the pastry starts to catch. The Plait is now ready to slice and serve.

TO FREEZE: Bring up the sides of the greaseproof paper to encase the Plait, then wrap in clingfilm. You can label the clingfilm or transfer the Plait to a large, labelled freezer bag and freeze flat for up to 1 month.

TO COOK FROM FROZEN: This can be cooked from frozen. Unwrap the Plait and place on a lined baking tray, then brush the top and sides with beaten egg and sprinkle over the sugar. Transfer to a 180°C/350°F/gas mark 4 oven and bake for 1 hour, covering with foil if the pastry starts to catch. The Plait is now ready to slice and serve.

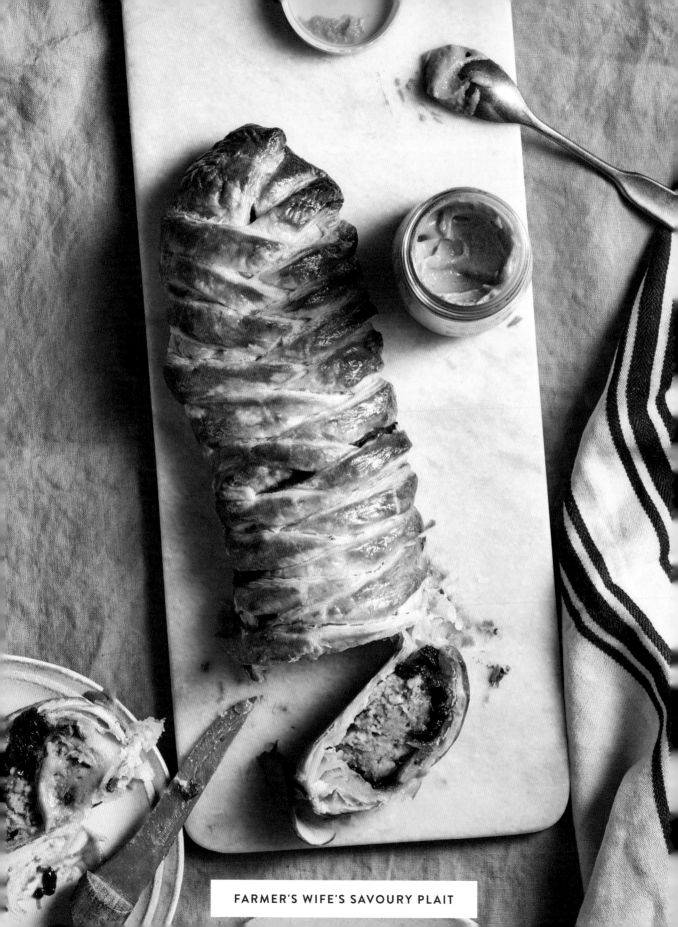

FARMER'S WIFE'S SAVOURY PLAIT

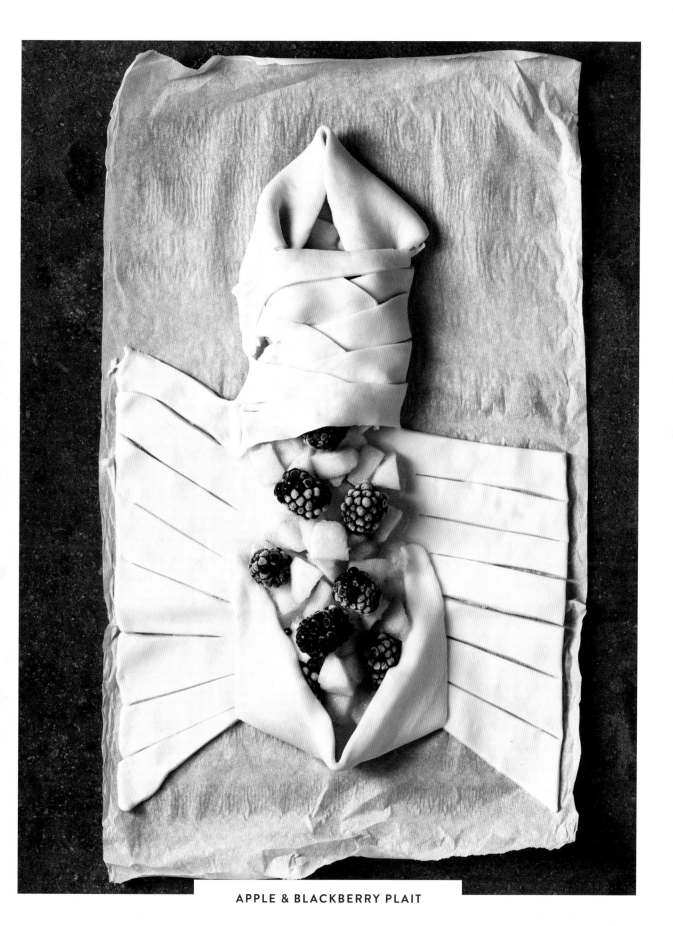

APPLE & BLACKBERRY PLAIT

BAKED SAUSAGE ZITI

PREP: 20 MINUTES
COOK: 45 MINUTES
SERVES 4

6 pork sausages
3 cups (300g) dried ziti
splash of olive oil
½ cup (60g) frozen,
  chopped onions
2 tsp frozen, chopped garlic
¼ cup (60g) bacon lardons
1 x 400g can chopped
  tomatoes
1 tsp dried Italian herb
  seasoning
½ cup (115g) ricotta cheese
1 cup (115g) grated
  mozzarella cheese
¼ cup (25g) grated
  Parmesan cheese

01 Preheat the oven to 180°C/350°F/gas mark 4 and line a baking tray with foil. Put the sausages on the prepared tray and transfer to the oven for 10–15 minutes, until cooked through.

02 While the sausages are cooking, place the pasta in a large pan and pour over boiling water to cover. Bring to the boil over a medium-high heat, then reduce to a simmer and cook according to packet instructions until just tender.

If you are also making the Baked Spinach Ziti, cook the pasta for that at the same time, ensuring you use a different pan.

03 While the pasta is cooking, heat a splash of olive oil in another pan over a medium heat, then add the onions, garlic, and bacon lardons and cook, stirring occasionally, until the lardons are crisp and golden. Add the tomatoes and Italian seasoning to the pan and stir to combine. Bring to the boil, then reduce to a gentle simmer while you prepare the other elements.

Make the sauce for the Spinach Ziti at the same time.

04 Drain and rinse the pasta, then place in a large baking dish. Slice the sausages into 1cm (½in) rounds, then add to the dish with the pasta. Pour over the sauce, then add all of the ricotta and half of the mozzarella cheese. Stir the mixture until really well combined, then scatter over the remaining mozzarella and all of the Parmesan cheese.

TO COOK: To cook straight away, simply transfer to an oven preheated to 180°C/350°F/gas mark 4 for 25–30 minutes, until golden and bubbling. Serve hot.

TO FREEZE: If you have space in your freezer, this can be left to cool, wrapped in a layer of clingfilm followed by a layer of foil, then frozen for up to 3 months. If you don't have space, omit the final sprinkling of cheese and, once cooled, transfer the mixture to a freezer bag and freeze flat.

TO COOK FROM FROZEN: This can be defrosted overnight in the fridge or cooked directly from frozen. If defrosting first, cook as described left, until golden and bubbling. If cooking from frozen, double the cooking time, covering with foil if the top starts to catch and ensuring the dish is piping hot before serving.

BAKED SPINACH ZITI

V

PREP: 20 MINUTES
COOK: 45 MINUTES
SERVES 4

3 cups (300g) dried ziti
splash of olive oil
½ cup (60g) frozen,
 chopped onions
2 tsp frozen, chopped garlic
1 x 400g can chopped
 tomatoes
1 tsp Italian herb seasoning
4 cups (180g) spinach
½ cup (115g) ricotta cheese
1 cup (115g) grated
 mozzarella cheese
¼ cup (25g) grated
 Parmesan cheese

This is a great meat-free comfort meal that can be made ahead to sit in your freezer, ready to pop straight in the oven after a busy day at work.

01 Place the pasta in a large pan and pour over boiling water to cover. Cook according to packet instructions until just tender.

02 While the pasta is cooking, heat a splash of olive oil in another pan over a medium heat, then add the onions and garlic and cook, stirring, for 1 minute, until softened. Add the tomatoes and Italian seasoning to the pan and stir to combine. Bring to the boil, then reduce to a gentle simmer while you prepare the other elements.

03 When the pasta is almost cooked, add the spinach to the pan and cook for one minute, until wilted, then drain and rinse the pasta and spinach through a colander.

04 Transfer the pasta and spinach mixture to a large baking dish. Pour over the sauce, then add all of the ricotta and half of the mozzarella cheese. Stir the mixture until really well combined, then scatter over the remaining mozzarella and all of the Parmesan cheese.

TO COOK: To cook straight away, simply transfer to an oven preheated to 180°C/350°F/ gas mark 4 for 25–30 minutes, until golden and bubbling. Serve hot.

TO FREEZE: If you have space in your freezer, this can be left to cool, then wrapped in a layer of clingfilm followed by a layer of foil, then frozen for up to 3 months. If you don't have space, omit the final sprinkling of cheese and, once cooled, transfer the mixture to a labelled freezer bag and freeze flat.

TO COOK FROM FROZEN: This can be defrosted overnight in the fridge or cooked directly from frozen. If defrosting first, cook as described left, until golden and bubbling. If cooking from frozen, double the cooking time, covering with foil if the top starts to catch and ensuring the dish is piping hot before serving.

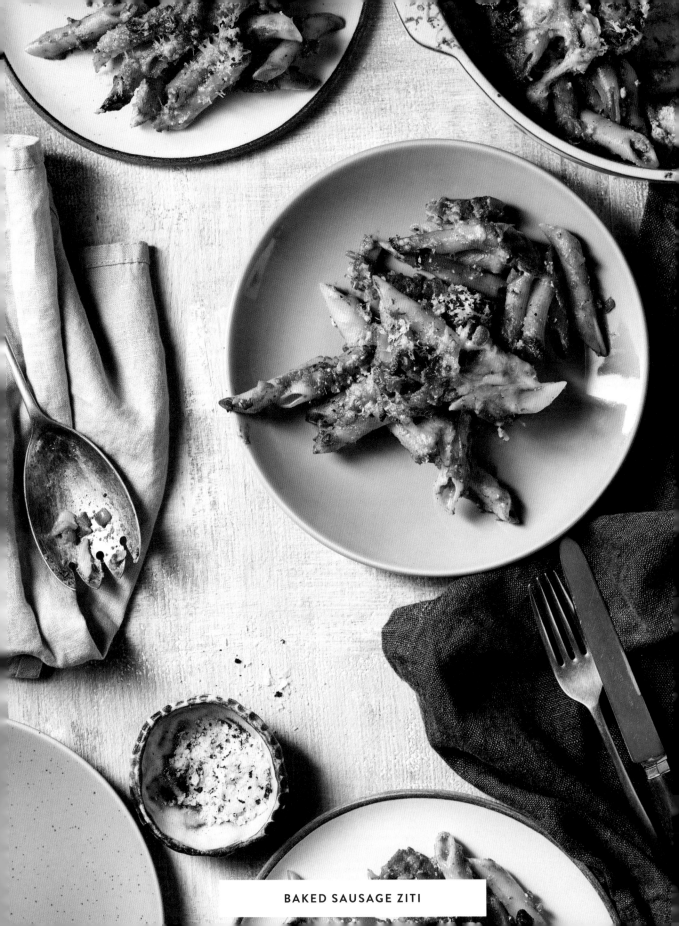

BAKED SAUSAGE ZITI

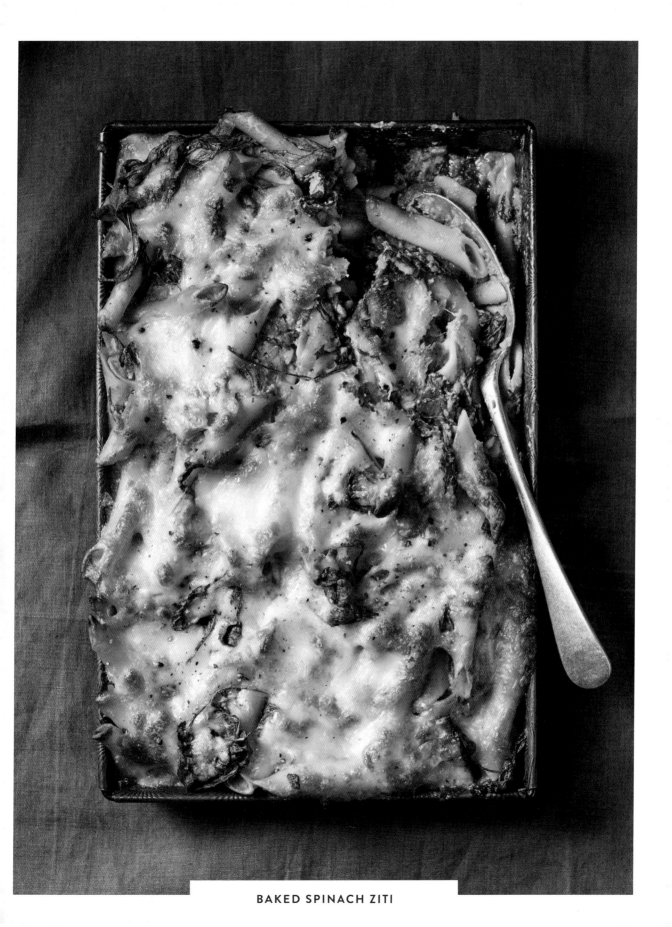

BAKED SPINACH ZITI

PEPPERONI CALZONES

PREP: 15 MINUTES
COOK: 15-20 MINUTES
**MAKES 2 LARGE
CALZONES, SERVING
4 PEOPLE**

2 x shop-bought, ready-
   rolled pizza doughs
2 cups (180g) grated
   mozzarella or cheddar
   cheese
1 cup (70g) chopped fresh
   mushrooms.
8–10 cherry tomatoes,
   halved
24 slices pepperoni
1 cup (240ml) Basic
   Tomato Sauce (p.200)
   or store-bought tomato
   sauce
1 egg, beaten

I love these two Calzone recipes because they are both so easy to make, yet feel like such a treat! They freeze brilliantly and can be cooked straight from frozen, so why not double or triple the recipe and make a few while you are at it?!

> If you are also making the sweet Calzones, make two neat piles of ingredients and set the three pizza doughs next to each other on the side, then you can simply assemble the separate fillings as you work through the recipes side-by-side.

01 Unroll both pizza doughs and set on your worktop, side-by-side. If the dough has a paper backing, leave that in place as it will make it easier to move around. If the dough doesn't have a paper backing, set on a lightly floured sheet of greaseproof paper.

02 Working on one half of each circle of dough, place ½ cup (45g) of the grated cheese on each pizza dough, followed by ½ cup (35g) mushrooms, half of the tomatoes, half of the pepperoni and then the remaining cheese. Finally, top each pile of ingredients with ½ cup (120ml) of the tomato sauce.

03 Brush a little of the egg wash around the edges, then bring the other half of the dough over the top of the filling to form a half-moon shape. Crimp the edges of the dough together to seal, then brush the top of each Calzone with a little beaten egg.

TO COOK: Slide the greaseproof paper onto a baking sheet and transfer to an oven preheated to 180°C/350°F/gas mark 4 for 15–20 minutes, until the Calzones are golden brown and the filling is bubbling. Let the calzones cool for a few minutes before serving, as the filling will be very hot.

TO FREEZE: Slide the Calzones onto a baking sheet then transfer to the freezer for a couple of hours to firm up. Once partially frozen and holding their shape, transfer the Calzones to a labelled freezer bag and freeze flat for up to 3 months.

TO COOK FROM FROZEN: The Calzones can be cooked straight from frozen. Simply place on a lined baking tray and cook in an oven preheated to 200°C/400°F/gas mark 6 for 30 minutes, until golden brown and the filling is piping hot.

BANANA, MARSHMALLOW & CHOCOLATE CALZONE

D

PREP: 15 MINUTES
COOK: 15-20 MINUTES
SERVES 4

1 x shop-bought, ready-
  rolled pizza dough
8 marshmallows
4 heaped tsp chocolate
  spread
2 bananas, sliced
1 egg, beaten
2 tsp caster sugar

01 Unroll the pizza dough and set on your worktop. If the dough has a paper backing, leave that in place as it will make it easier to move around. If the dough doesn't have a paper backing, set on a lightly floured sheet of greaseproof paper. Set aside.

02 Place a generous teaspoon of chocolate spread on one of the marshmallows, then sandwich together with another marshmallow. Repeat, until all of the marshmallows and chocolate spread have been used up.

03 Lay the banana slices on one half of the circle of dough, then lay the four marshmallow-and-chocolate sandwiches over the top. Brush a little of the egg wash around the edges, then bring the other half of the dough over the top of the filling to form a half-moon shape. Crimp the edges of the dough together to seal, then brush the top of the calzone with a little beaten egg and sprinkle over the caster sugar.

TO COOK: Slide the greaseproof paper onto a baking sheet and transfer to an oven preheated to 180°C/350°F/gas mark 4 for 15–20 minutes, until the Calzone is golden brown and the filling is bubbling. Let the Calzone cool for a few minutes before serving, as the filling will be very hot.

TO FREEZE: Slide the Calzone onto a baking sheet then transfer to the freezer for a couple of hours to firm up. Once partially frozen and holding their shape, transfer the Calzone to a labelled freezer bag and freeze flat for up to 3 months.

TO COOK FROM FROZEN: The Calzone can be cooked straight from frozen. Simply place on a lined baking tray and cook in an oven preheated to 200°C/400°F/gas mark 6 for 30 minutes, until golden brown and the filling is piping hot.

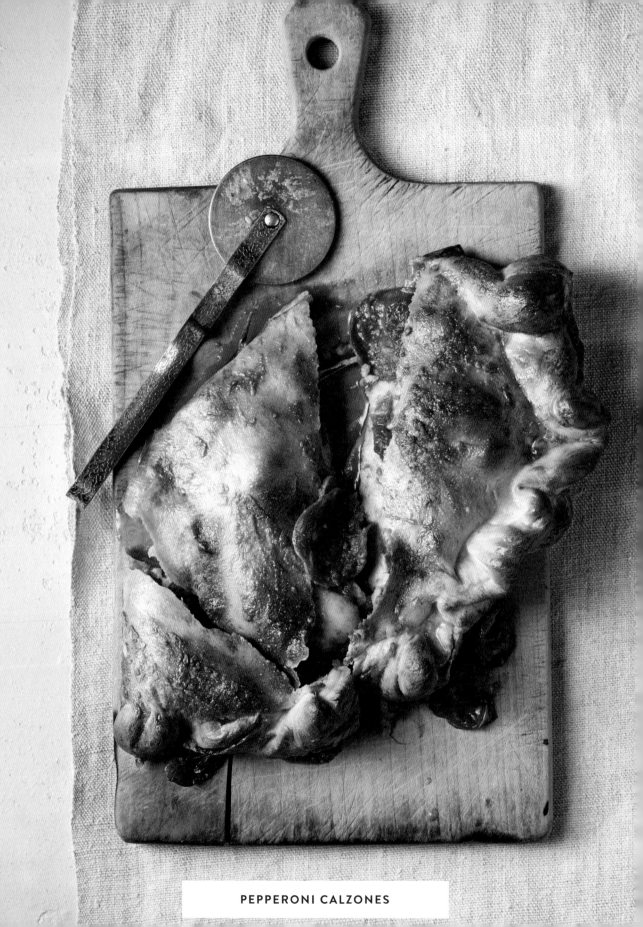

PEPPERONI CALZONES

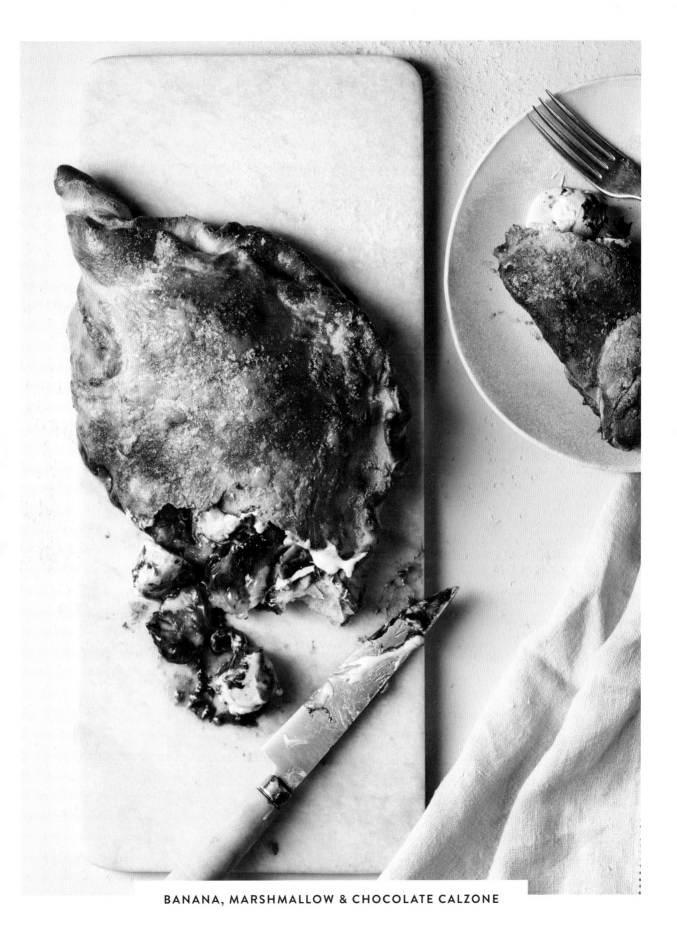

BANANA, MARSHMALLOW & CHOCOLATE CALZONE

MOUSSAKA

PREP: 20 MINS
COOK: 1 HR
SERVES 6

butter, for greasing
splash of olive oil
1 cup (115g) frozen,
   chopped onions
2 tsp frozen, chopped garlic
500g minced lamb
2 x 400g cans whole
   tomatoes, drained
2 tbsp tomato purée
1 tbsp dried mixed Italian
   herbs
1 tsp ground cinnamon
500g frozen, roasted
   aubergines
1 x 250g tub ricotta cheese
1 x 200g pack feta cheese
1 large egg, beaten
salt and freshly ground
   pepper, to taste

01 Grease a large baking dish with butter.
02 Heat a splash of oil in a large pan, then add the onions, garlic and minced lamb and cook, stirring continuously, for 5–7 minutes over a medium heat, until the meat has browned. Drain any excess fat from the pan then add the tomatoes, tomato purée, dried herbs and cinnamon and stir to combine. Reduce the heat to a simmer and leave to cook for 20 minutes.

While the meat is simmering, make the Lamb & Feta Burgers.

03 Using scissors, snip the frozen aubergine slices into 2.5cm (1in) strips and layer half of these in the base of your prepared dish. Set aside.
04 In a large bowl, beat together the ricotta, feta and beaten egg until well combined, then season generously with salt and pepper.
05 Once the meat has finished simmering, pour the mixture into the baking dish over the layer of aubergines, ensuring that it reaches the edges in an even layer. Top the meat with another layer of aubergines, then pour the cheese and egg mixture over the top and spread to form an even layer.

TO COOK: Transfer to an oven preheated to 180°C/350°F/ gas mark 4 for 35–40 minutes, until golden and bubbling. If the top of the Moussaka browns too quickly, cover with foil for the remainder of the cooking time.

TO FREEZE: If you are making the Moussaka ahead to freeze, set aside until cooled to room temperature, then cover with a layer of clingfilm followed by a layer of foil. Label clearly and transfer to the freezer for up to 1 month.

TO COOK FROM FROZEN: Remove the Moussaka from the freezer and defrost thoroughly, then cook the Moussaka as described in the *To Cook* section, left.

LAMB & FETA BURGERS

PREP: 5 MINS
COOK: 12 MINS
MAKES 4 LARGE OR 6 MEDIUM BURGERS

500g minced lamb
2 tbsp Worcestershire
  sauce
2 tsp dried rosemary
2 tsp dried thyme
100g feta cheese, cut into
  1cm (½in) cubes
splash of olive oil, for frying
salt and freshly ground
  pepper, to taste
To Serve:
4 brioche burger buns,
  halved
salad leaves
corn on the cob
sauce if your choice
  (sriracha mayo or
  cucumber yogurt would
  work well)

These are so easy to make and are frozen raw, so the minute you've divided up your patties, you're moving on to the next meal. I freeze these with brioche burger buns and corn on the cob alongside, so my whole meal is ready to pull out of the freezer and defrost in one go.

01 Put the meat, Worcestershire sauce, dried herbs and a generous grinding of salt and pepper in a large bowl and mix with your fingers until well combined.

02 Depending on the size you want your burgers, split the mixture in four or six equal-sized portions, then divide the cubed feta evenly between the portions of meat. Shape each portion of meat into a burger patty, pressing the feta cubes firmly into the mixture.

If you are making the Moussaka, return to step 3 now.

Zhuzh it Up!
For a grown-up twist, add some finely chopped fennel tops to the burger mixture to give a delicious hint of anise.

TO COOK: To cook the Burgers, heat a splash of olive oil in a frying pan over a medium heat, then cook for 5–6 minutes on each side, until cooked through. Serve in brioche buns with salad, corn on the cob and your choice of sauce alongside.

TO FREEZE: Transfer to a clearly labelled freezer bag in a single layer, then freeze flat for up to 1 month.

TO COOK FROM FROZEN: These are best defrosted and cooked in a pan as described left. If you want to cook them from frozen, cook in an oven preheated to 200°C/400°F/ gas mark 6 for 25–30 minutes, turning halfway through.

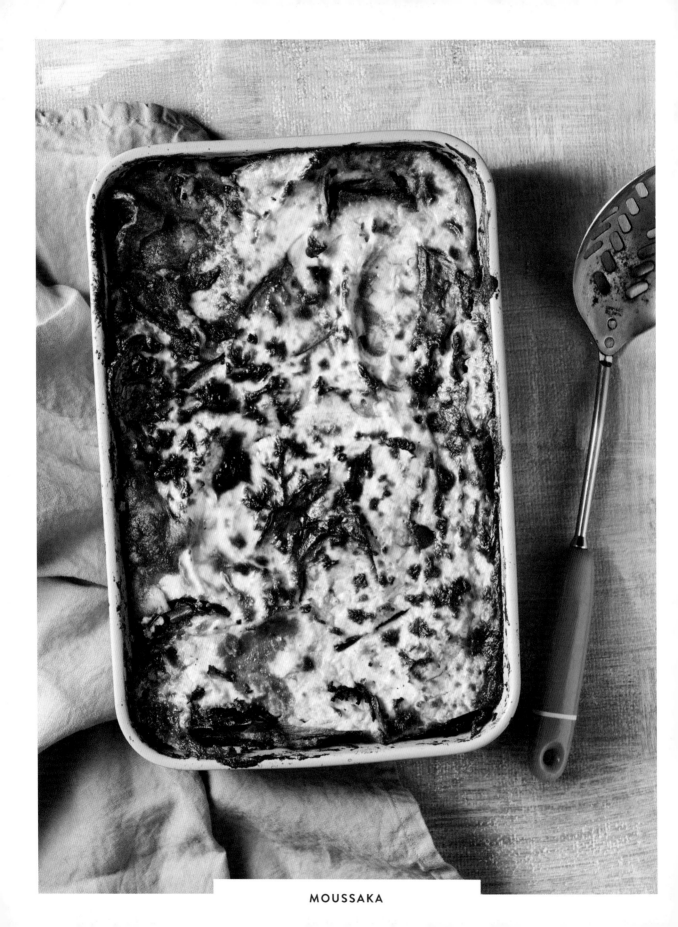

MOUSSAKA

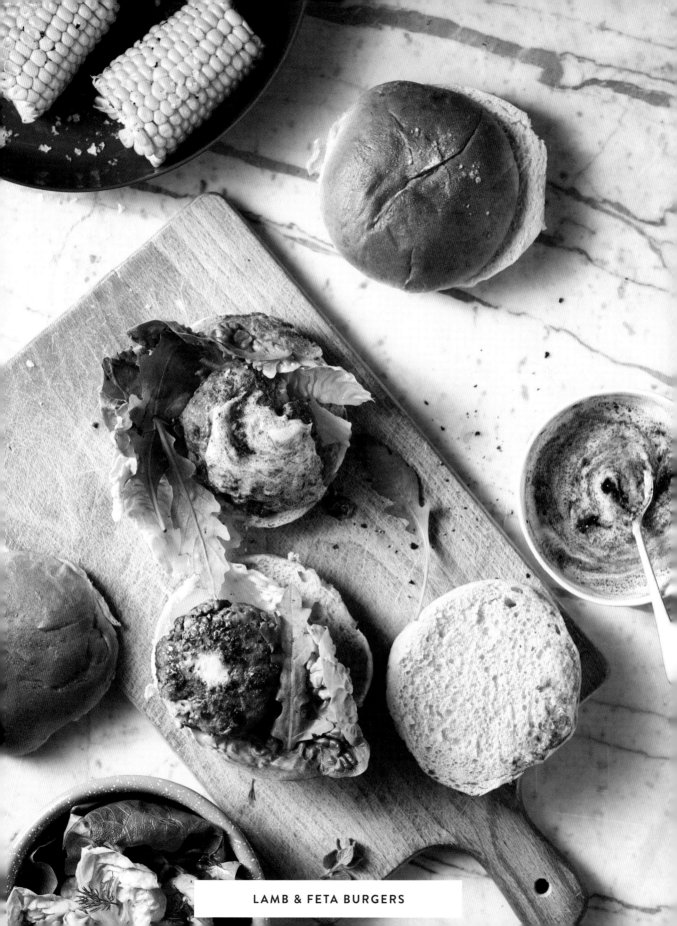

LAMB & FETA BURGERS

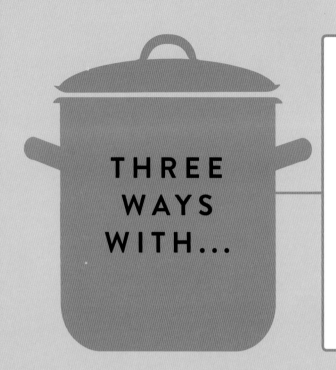

THREE WAYS WITH...

LAMB & FETA BURGERS

Now that you've prepared your Lamb & Feta Burgers, what are you going to do with them? Below are three simple ideas for different ways of serving them that will keep mealtimes feeling fresh and different every time!

LAMB & FETA BURGERS IN BUNS WITH WEDGES

4 Lamb & Feta Burgers (p.87)
4 brioche burger buns
splash of olive oil
2 onions, finely sliced
2 beef tomatoes, sliced
4 lettuce leaves
frozen potato wedges, to serve

01 Cook the potato wedges in the oven according to packet instructions and prepare and cook the Lamb & Feta Burgers according to instructions on page 87.

02 Heat a splash of olive oil in a frying pan over a medium heat, then add the sliced onions and cook, stirring occasionally, for 10–15 minutes, until soft and starting to turn golden.

03 To assemble, place the burgers inside the buns and top with the fried onions, lettuce leaves and tomato slices. Serve hot with the cooked wedges alongside.

LAMB & FETA MEATBALLS

Lamb & Feta Burger mix (p.87)
1 x 400g pack Mediterranean
  roasting vegetables
splash of olive oil
2⅓ cups (400g) couscous
2⅓ cups (560ml) chicken stock
1 handful chopped fresh
  coriander

01 Make the Lamb & Feta Burger mix according
    to the instructions on page 87, but rather
    than shaping into patties at the end of step 2,
    divide the mixture into 12 equal-size pieces
    and form each into a ball shape.
02 Preheat the oven to 180°C/350°F/gas mark
    4. Spread the roasting vegetables over a
    baking tray and drizzle over a splash of olive
    oil. Transfer to the oven and cook for
    15 minutes, then add the meatballs to
    the tray and cook for another 15 minutes,
    turning them once, until the meatballs are
    cooked through and the vegetables are crisp
    and tender.
03 While the meatballs and vegetables are
    cooking, prepare the couscous by bringing the
    stock to the boil in a pan, then pouring in the
    couscous and removing the pan from the heat.
    Stir once, then set the pan aside, covered, for
    5 minutes. Fluff the couscous up with a fork
    and set aside.
04 Once cooked, spoon the roasted vegetables
    into the pan with the couscous and stir to
    combine. Divide the couscous between 4
    plates, then spoon over the meatballs. Serve
    hot, garnished with fresh coriander leaves.

LAMB & FETA PITTAS
WITH BEETROOT SALAD

4 Lamb & Feta Burgers (p.87)
4 pitta breads
4 tbsp mayonnaise (optional)
1 x 300g pack store-bought
  beetroot salad
mixed salad leaves
1 red onion, sliced
2 tomatoes, sliced

01 Prepare and cook the Lamb & Feta Burgers
    according to instructions on page 87.
02 While the burgers are cooking, toast the pitta
    breads then slice open, being careful of any
    escaping steam as you do.
03 Spread the inside of each pitta with a
    tablespoon of mayonnaise, if using, then add
    a spoonful of beetroot salad, some salad
    leaves and a few slices of onion and tomato.
    Finally, add a cooked burger to each pitta and
    serve hot.

PULLED PORK

(M)

PREP: 20 MINUTES
COOK: 8–10 HOURS
SERVES 6–9

1 tbsp brown sugar
½ tsp ground cumin
½ tsp ground cinnamon
1 tbsp chilli powder
1 x 1.8–2.25kg boneless
   shoulder of pork
2½ cups (290g) frozen,
   chopped onions
3 tsp frozen, chopped
   garlic
1 cup (240ml) chicken
   stock
2 cups (480ml) store-
   bought barbecue sauce

There's no getting round the fact that this needs a long time in the oven, but the prep is minimal and the result is so delicious that it is more than worth the effort. A large pork shoulder will yield loads of meat, so one long cook will easily fill your freezer with enough deliciously juicy pork for several meals.

01 Preheat the oven to 110°C/230°F/gas mark ¼.

02 Put the sugar, cumin, cinnamon and chilli powder in a bowl and mix to combine, then rub this mixture over the pork shoulder, covering all of the meat but avoiding the fat. Set aside.

03 Put the onions, garlic and stock in the base of a lidded casserole dish large enough to fit your pork and stir to combine. Add the pork to the dish, fat-side up and cover with the lid, or, if your dish does not have a lid, cover with foil.

04 Transfer the pork to the oven to cook for 8–10 hours, until the pork is unctuous, juicy and falling apart and the internal temperature reads 90°C/194°F when checked with a meat thermometer or temperature probe.

If you are also making the Pulled Lamb recipe (p.98), marinate the lamb and put it in the fridge now so that the flavours can develop while the pork is in the oven.

05 Transfer the cooked pork to a chopping board and use a slotted spoon to transfer the onions into a bowl. Set the casserole aside until the stock and juices have cooled completely, then spoon away any fat that has collected on top of the liquid.

Increase the oven temperature for the lamb now, then pop it in the oven while you finish preparing the pork.

06 Slice away and discard the top layer of fat from the cooked pork shoulder, then use two forks to 'pull' or shred the pork, discarding any pieces that are very fatty. Transfer the pulled pork to a large bowl and add the barbecue sauce, cooked onions and 1½ cups (360ml) of the cooled cooking liquid, then stir everything to combine. The pork should be very moist.

TO SERVE: The pork is now ready to serve. It is delicious served in brioche buns with corn on the cob on the side.

TO FREEZE: Portion the pork out into large, labelled freezer bags. I serve ½ cup of pulled pork per person, so 2 cups of the mixture is perfect for a family of four. Freeze the bags flat for up to 3 months.

TO COOK FROM FROZEN: Remove a bag of Pulled Pork from the freezer and allow to defrost fully in the fridge. Once defrosted, simply heat in the microwave for 3–4 minutes, or transfer to a baking dish and cook in an oven preheated to 180°C/350°F/gas mark 4 for 10–15 minutes.

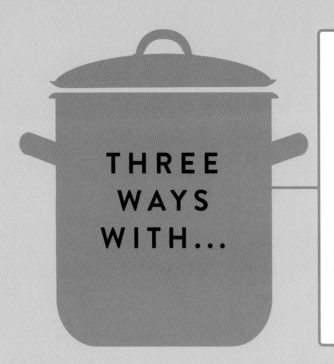

THREE WAYS WITH...

PULLED PORK

Now that you've prepared your Pulled Pork, what are you going to do with it? Below are three simple ideas for different ways of serving it that will keep mealtimes feeling fresh and different every time.

BAKED SWEET POTATOES WITH PULLED PORK

4 Made-in-advance Baked
   Sweet Potatoes (p.193)
4 portions (2 cups) Pulled Pork
   (p.92), defrosted if frozen
1 x 200g can sweetcorn,
   drained
small bunch spring onions, sliced
1 cup (90g) cheddar cheese
mixed salad leaves, to serve

01 Remove the sweet potatoes from the freezer, place on a baking sheet and reheat in the oven at 200°C/400°F/gas mark 6 for 10–15 minutes, until crisp. Put the Pulled Pork, sweetcorn and spring onions in a baking dish and stir to combine, then place in the oven for the same time as the potatoes.

02 Once reheated, slice open the potatoes and divide between four serving plates. Top each potato with a cupful of the Pulled Pork mixture and sprinkle over the grated cheese. Serve the potatoes with the mixed salad leaves alongside.

PULLED PORK & APPLE BUNS

4 portions (2 cups) Pulled Pork
  (p.92), defrosted if frozen
4 brioche burger buns
4 tbsp apple sauce
1 apple, peeled and thinly sliced
mixed salad leaves, to serve

01 Transfer the Pulled Pork to a heatproof bowl
    and cook in the microwave for 2–3 minutes,
    until piping hot.
02 Slice open the buns and fill each with a cupful
    of the Pulled Pork, then top with a tablespoon
    of the apple sauce and a couple of slices of
    sliced apple. Serve the buns with a mixed salad
    alongside.

PULLED PORK QUESADILLAS

4 portions (2 cups) Pulled Pork
  (p.92), defrosted if frozen
8 tortilla wraps
spray oil, for cooking the
  quesadillas
sliced jalapenos (optional)
2 cups (180g) grated cheddar
  cheese
store-bought guacamole, salsa
  and sour cream, to serve

01 Transfer the Pulled Pork to a heatproof bowl
    and cook in the microwave for 2–3 minutes,
    until piping hot. Warm the tortilla wraps in the
    microwave for 20 seconds.
02 Place a large frying pan over a medium heat
    and add a couple sprays of oil, then add one
    of the wraps to the pan. Spoon 2 tablespoons
    of the Pulled Pork onto one half of the wrap,
    then scatter over some grated cheese and
    jalapenos, if using.
03 Fold over the wrap to form a half-moon shape
    and flatten down slightly with a spatula, then
    flip so that both sides of the quesadilla are just
    golden brown. Set aside, while you make the
    remaining quesadillas.
04 Once all the quesadillas are cooked, cut in
    half and serve with guacamole, salsa and sour
    cream alongside for dipping.

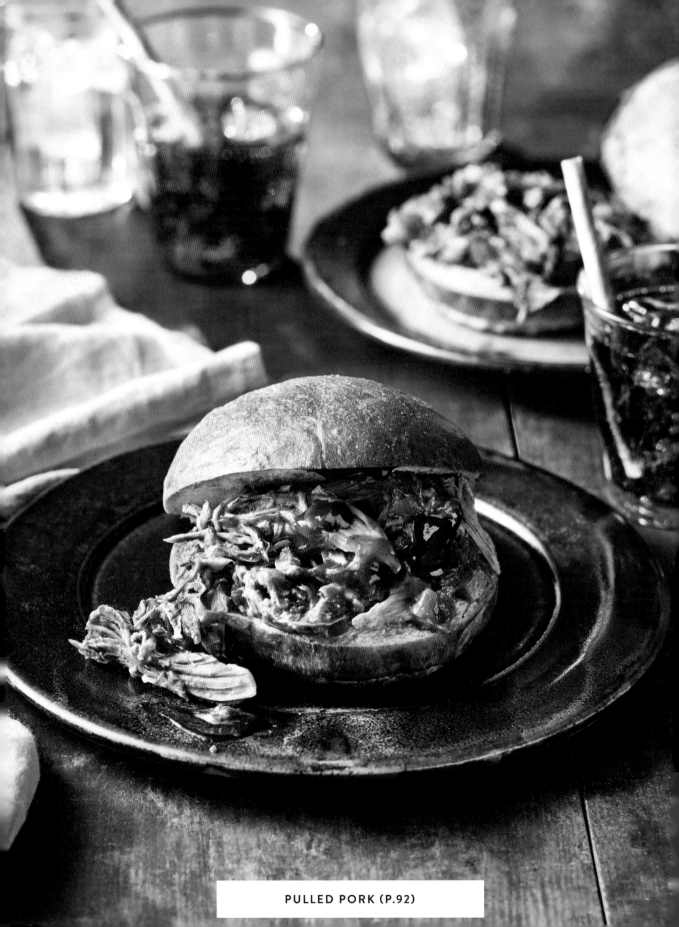

PULLED PORK (P.92)

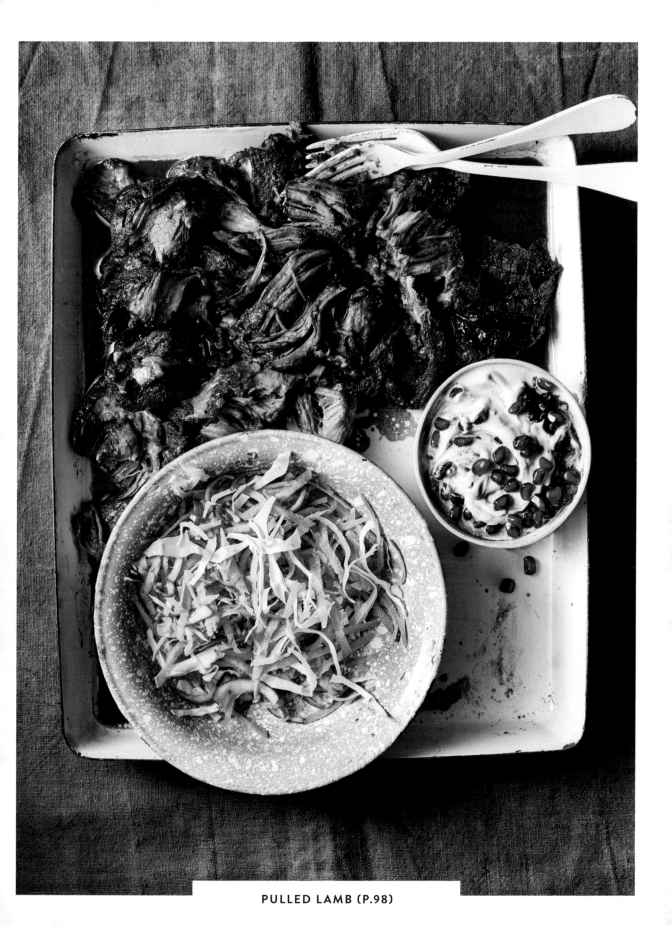

PULLED LAMB (P.98)

PULLED LAMB

(M)

PREP: 20 MINUTES
COOK: 5 HOURS
SERVES 6-9

1 tbsp brown sugar
2½ tsp ground cumin
2½ tsp ground cinnamon
4 tbsp lemon juice (for
   ease, I use store-bought)
1 x 1.8–2.25kg boneless
   shoulder of lamb
2 cups (480ml)
   pomegranate juice
1 x 500g bag frozen, sliced
   red onions
4 tsp frozen, chopped
   garlic
3 tbsp olive oil
2 cups (480ml)
   pomegranate molasses
2 tbsp runny honey

This is such a delicious and versatile dish. Kids love it served in fluffy bread rolls, but it also makes a great dinner-party dish when dressed up with pomegranate seeds and served with flatbreads, tzatziki and couscous alongside.

01 Preheat the oven to 170°C/325°F/gas mark 3.

02 Put the sugar, cumin, cinnamon and lemon juice in a bowl and stir to form a paste, then rub the mixture all over the lamb.

If you are making this while the Pulled Pork (p.92) is in the oven, transfer the lamb to the fridge to marinate now, while the pork finishes cooking. This isn't essential, but will yield a better end flavour.

03 Put the pomegranate juice, sliced red onions and garlic in the base of a lidded casserole dish large enough to fit your lamb and stir to combine. Add the lamb to the dish, skin-side up and cover with the lid, or, if your dish does not have a lid, cover with foil.

04 Transfer the lamb to the oven to cook for approximately 5 hours, until the lamb is unctuous, juicy and falling apart and the internal temperature reads 90°C/194°F when checked with a meat thermometer or temperature probe.

05 20 minutes before the lamb is due out of the oven, combine the olive oil and 1 cup (240ml) of the pomegranate molasses in a bowl and brush over the meat. Return the lamb to the oven, uncovered, for the last 20 minutes.

06 Transfer the cooked lamb to a chopping board and use a slotted spoon to transfer the onions into a bowl.

07 Pour the cooking liquid from the lamb into a small pan along with the honey and the remaining 1 cup (240ml) of pomegranate molasses. Place over a high heat and cook, stirring occasionally, for about 5 minutes, until reduced and thickened.

08 Slice away and discard any fat from the cooked lamb shoulder, then use two forks to 'pull' or shred the lamb, discarding any pieces that are very fatty. Transfer the meat to a large bowl with the cooked onions and the thickened cooking liquid, then stir everything to combine. The lamb should be very moist.

TO SERVE: The lamb is now ready to serve. It is delicious served in brioche buns or with flatbreads and tzatziki.

TO FREEZE: Portion the lamb out into large, labelled freezer bags. I serve ½ cup of pulled lamb per person, so 2 cups of the mixture is perfect for a family of four. Freeze the bags flat for up to 3 months.

TO COOK FROM FROZEN: Remove a bag of Pulled Lamb from the freezer and allow to defrost fully in the fridge. Once defrosted, simply heat in the microwave for 3–4 minutes, or transfer to a baking dish and cook in an oven preheated to 180°C/350°F/gas mark 4 for 10–15 minutes.

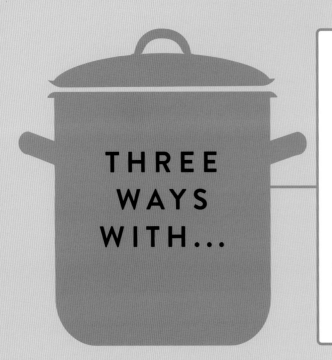

THREE WAYS WITH...

PULLED LAMB

Now that you've prepared your Pulled Lamb, what are you going to do with it? Below are three simple ideas for different ways of serving it that will keep mealtimes feeling fresh and different every time!

PULLED LAMB & POMEGRANATE SALAD FLATBREADS

3–4 portions (about 2 cups) Pulled Lamb (p.98 – you don't need much for this recipe, so this is perfect if you have a small batch left in the freezer)

4–6 store-bought flatbreads

shredded lettuce

3 tomatoes, sliced

½ red onion, finely sliced

½ cup (120ml) natural yogurt

4 tbsp pomegranate seeds

01 If you have defrosted the lamb, warm it through in an oven preheated to 180°C/350°F/gas mark 4 for 15 minutes, adding the flatbreads to the oven for the last 5 minutes of cooking time.

02 Once warmed, slice open the flatbreads and add a bed of lettuce, tomatoes and onion to each. Divide the lamb between the flatbreads, then add a spoonful of yogurt and a scattering of pomegranate seeds to each. Serve.

PULLED LAMB WITH GREEN BEANS & DAUPHINOISE POTATOES

4 portions (2 cups) Pulled Lamb
  (p.98)
½ quantity Potato Dauphinoise
  (p.196)
1 x 200–225g pack green
  beans
store-bought redcurrant jelly,
  to serve

01 If you have defrosted the lamb and potatoes, warm them through in an oven preheated to 180°C/350°F/gas mark 4 for 15 minutes, otherwise prepare and cook as per the recipes on pages 98 and 196.

02 While the lamb and potatoes are warming, cook the green beans in a pan of boiling water until tender, but still retaining some bite.

03 Divide the lamb, potatoes and green beans between four serving plates and serve hot with the redcurrant jelly alongside.

PULLED LAMB WITH COUSCOUS SALAD

4 portions (2 cups) Pulled Lamb
  (p.98)
2 x 100g packs microwave
  Mediterranean couscous
8 cherry tomatoes, halved
½ red onion, finely chopped
100g feta cheese, crumbled
  (optional)
handful chopped fresh
  coriander

01 If you have defrosted the lamb, warm it through in an oven preheated to 180°C/350°F/gas mark 4 for 15 minutes.

02 While the lamb is warming in the oven, cook the couscous in the microwave according to the packet instructions, then pour into a bowl with the cherry tomatoes, red onion and feta cheese, if using.

03 Divide the couscous between four serving plates, then spoon over the lamb. Serve hot, garnished with fresh coriander.

LAZY LASAGNE

PREP: 15 MINUTES
COOK: 65 MINUTES
SERVES 4–6

splash of olive oil
1 cup (115g) frozen,
    chopped onions
1 tsp frozen, chopped garlic
500g minced beef
1 cup (70g) shop-bought
    grated carrot or 1 cup
    (70g) frozen, chopped
    mushrooms (optional)
1 x 500g carton passata
2 tablespoons tomato purée
2 x 400g cans chopped
    tomatoes
3 tsp dried oregano
6 dried lasagne sheets
3 large mozzarella balls,
    shredded
2 x 250g tubs ricotta
    cheese

01 Heat the oil in a large pan over a medium heat, then add the onions and garlic and cook for 1 minute, stirring continuously. Add the beef to the pan, breaking up with a wooden spoon, and cook, stirring occasionally, until browned.

While the beef is browning, make the Meatballs

02 Once the beef has browned, add the carrot or mushrooms (if using), passata, tomato purée, chopped tomatoes and oregano and stir to combine. Leave the mixture to cook over a medium-high heat until thickened.

03 While the sauce is thickening, make the cheese layer by combining the mozzarella and ricotta in a large bowl and stirring until well combined.

04 To assemble the lasagne place 1½–2 cups of the meat mixture in the base of your dish, topping with two of the dried lasagne sheets. Spread a thin layer of the cheese mixture over the top of the pasta, then repeat the layers until you reach the top of the dish, ensuring that you finish with a layer of the cheese mixture.

Note
For an even simpler lasagne, replace the sauce ingredients with 2 x 600g jars (about 4 cups) of store-bought tomato sauce.

TO COOK: Simply place in an oven preheated to 190°C/375°F/gas mark 5 for 45 minutes, until beautifully golden brown and bubbling.

TO FREEZE: If you are making this ahead to freeze, set aside to cool to room temperature then cover the dish, either with a plastic lid or with a layer of clingfilm followed by a layer of foil, then label and transfer to the freezer for up to 3 months.

TO COOK FROM FROZEN: This can be defrosted overnight in the fridge or cooked from frozen. If defrosting first, cook the lasagne as described left. If cooking from frozen, cook at the same temperature, increasing the time to 1¼–1½ hours and ensuring the dish is piping hot before serving.

MOZZARELLA STUFFED MEATBALLS

PREP: 15 MINUTES
COOK: 30 MINUTES
MAKES 16 MEATBALLS, SERVING 4 PEOPLE

500g minced beef
½ cup (60g) dried breadcrumbs
1 egg, beaten
2 tsp dried oregano
1 tsp frozen, chopped garlic
1 tbsp Worcestershire sauce
1 x 210g tub mozzarella pearls
1 quantity Basic Tomato Sauce (p.200) or 1 large jar store-bought tomato sauce
pasta of your choice, to serve
grated Parmesan cheese, to serve

These meatballs, with a deliciously gooey mozzarella filling, are cooked before freezing, then simply defrosted and quickly reheated on the day you want to serve them.

01 Preheat the oven to 180°C/350°F/gas mark 4 and line a large baking tray with foil.

02 Put the minced beef, breadcrumbs, egg, oregano, garlic and Worcester sauce in a large bowl and mix together with your hands until well combined.

03 To form the meatballs, divide the meat mixture into four equal-sized portions, then divide each portion into four again. Using your hands, gently flatten each piece of meat and place a mozzarella pearl in the centre, then form the meatball around the mozzarella, rolling in the palms of your hands to create a ball shape.

04 Place the Meatballs on the prepared baking tray, transfer to the oven and cook for 15 minutes, until golden and cooked all the way through.

TO COOK: Heat the tomato sauce in a pan until bubbling and cook the pasta in a separate pan according to packet instructions. Divide the pasta between serving plates and top with the Meatballs, then spoon over the tomato sauce. Serve hot, sprinkled with freshly grated Parmesan.

TO FREEZE: Set the cooked Meatballs aside until cooled to room temperature, then transfer to a labelled freezer bag along with the sauce. Freeze flat for up to 3 months.

TO COOK FROM FROZEN: Defrost fully in the fridge. Put the defrosted Meatballs and sauce in a large pan over a medium-high heat and leave to cook for about 15 minutes, until the sauce is bubbling and the Meatballs are piping hot all the way through. Serve as described in the *To Cook* section, left.

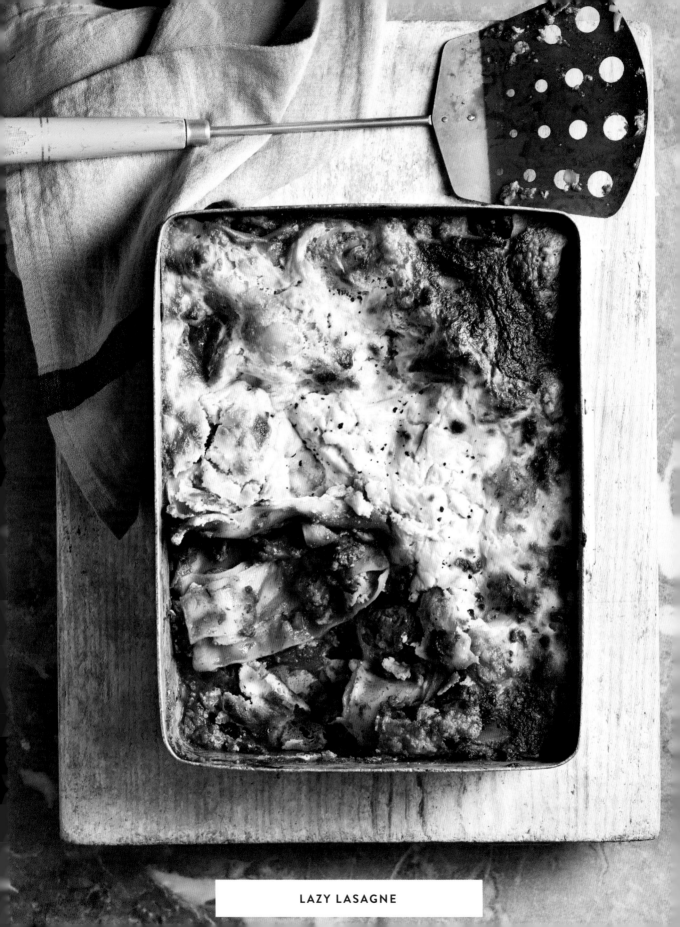

LAZY LASAGNE

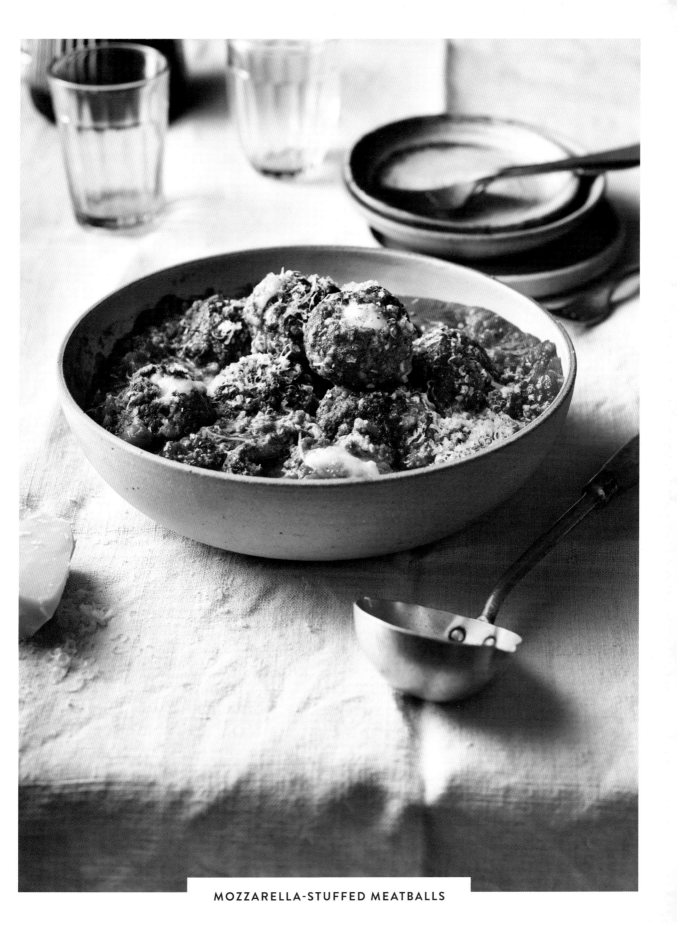

MOZZARELLA-STUFFED MEATBALLS

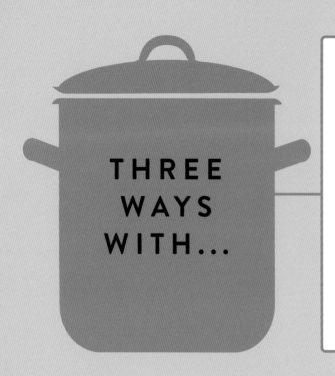

THREE WAYS WITH...

MOZZARELLA -STUFFED MEATBALLS

Now that you've prepared your Mozzarella-stuffed Meatballs, what are you going to do with them? Below are three simple ideas for different ways of serving them that will keep mealtimes feeling fresh and different every time!

SPAGHETTI & MEATBALLS

1 x quantity Mozzarella-stuffed
  Meatballs (p.103)
400g spaghetti
grated Parmesan cheese,
  to serve

01 Simply prepare and cook the Meatballs as per the recipe on page 103. While the Meatballs are in the oven, cook the pasta in a pan of boiling water according to pack instructions.

02 Drain and rinse the spaghetti through a colander, then divide between serving plates and spoon the Meatballs and tomato sauce over. Scatter over some grated Parmesan and serve hot.

MOZZARELLA MEATBALL SUBS

1 x quantity Mozzarella-stuffed
  Meatballs (p.103)
4 submarine rolls
shredded lettuce, to serve
  (optional)
2–3 tomatoes, sliced
grated cheese, to serve
  (optional)

01 Prepare and cook the Meatballs as per the
    recipe on page 103. While the Meatballs are
    in the oven slice open the submarine rolls and
    prepare the rest of your fillings.
02 Once cooked, remove the Meatballs from
    the sauce and cut in half. Leave the sauce on
    the heat for 5–10 minutes to thicken further.
03 Put a bed of lettuce, if using, and a few slices
    of tomatoes in each roll, then divide the
    halved Meatballs between each roll. Spoon
    over the thickened tomato sauce and top with
    grated cheese, if using.

MOZZARELLA MEATBALL SALAD

1 x quantity Mozzarella-stuffed
  Meatballs (p.103)
4 tomatoes, sliced
salad leaves and any other items
  that you want to add (I like
  sweetcorn, cucumber and
  spring onions)
store-bought ranch dressing, to
  serve (optional)

If, like me, you occasionally try and avoid eating
too many carbs or wheat, this is a great, lighter
option that means that you still get to enjoy the
oozy deliciousness of the Meatballs.

01 Prepare and cook the Meatballs as per the
    recipe on page 103. While the Meatballs are in
    the oven prepare your salad.
02 To serve, simply plate up the salad and spoon
    the Meatballs over. Serve with ranch dressing
    alongside.

COTTAGE PIE WITH ROOT VEGETABLES

PREP: 15 MINUTES
COOK: 40 MINUTES
SERVES 4

2 tbsp olive oil
1 cup (115g) frozen,
    chopped onions
1 cup (115g) frozen, sliced
    carrots
500g beef mince
1 beef stock cube
1 x 400g can chopped
    tomatoes
2 tbsp tomato purée or
    ketchup
1 cup (60g) button
    mushrooms, halved
2 x 425g packs pre-cooked
    root vegetable mash

If you are also making the Shepherd's Pie, lay out the ingredients for both recipes and work with two pans alongside each other on the hob. The stages are very similar, so it is very easy to make both dishes at the same time.

01 Heat the oil in a large pan over a medium-high heat, then add the onions and carrots and cook, stirring continuously, for 2–3 minutes, until softened. Add the beef mince to the pan and crumble over the stock cube, then cook, stirring to break up the mince, until browned, about 5 minutes.

02 Add the chopped tomatoes and tomato purée or paste and mix well to combine, then reduce the heat to a simmer and leave to cook for 10 minutes.

03 Add the mushrooms to the pan, then stir until well combined. Spoon the beef mixture into the base of large baking dish, spoon over the root vegetable mash then spread over the top with a spatula or palette knife to form an even layer.

TO SERVE: Bake in an oven preheated to 180°C/350°F/gas mark 4 for 20–30 minutes, until piping hot all the way through. Serve hot with your choice of vegetables alongside.

TO FREEZE: Leave until completely cooled, then cover the dish, either with a plastic lid or with a layer of clingfilm followed by a layer of foil, then label and transfer to the freezer for up to 3 months.

TO COOK FROM FROZEN: This can be defrosted overnight in the fridge or cooked directly from frozen. If defrosting first, cook as described left, until golden and bubbling. If cooking from frozen, increase the cooking time to 1 hour 10 minutes, covering with foil if the top starts to catch and ensuring a knife inserted into the centre is piping hot before serving.

SHEPHERD'S PIE WITH SWEET POTATO MASH

PREP: 15 MINUTES
COOK: 40 MINUTES
SERVES 4

2 tablespoons olive oil
1 cup (115g) frozen, chopped onions
1 cup (115g) frozen, sliced carrots
500g lamb mince
1 lamb stock cube
1 x 400g can chopped tomatoes
½ tsp dried rosemary
2 tbsp redcurrant jelly
1 cup (155g) frozen peas
2 x 425g packs pre-cooked sweet potato mash

01 Heat the oil in a large pan over a medium-high heat, then add the onions and carrots and cook, stirring continuously, for 2–3 minutes, until softened. Add the lamb mince to the pan and crumble over the stock cube, then cook, stirring to break up the mince, until browned, about 5 minutes.

02 Add the chopped tomatoes, dried rosemary and redcurrant jelly to the pan and mix well to combine, then reduce the heat to a simmer and leave to cook for 10 minutes.

03 Add the peas to the pan, then stir through the mixture until well combined. Spoon the lamb mixture into the base of large baking dish, spoon over the sweet potato mash then spread over the top with a spatula or palette knife to form an even layer.

TO SERVE: Bake in an oven preheated to 180°C/350°F/gas mark 4 for 20–30 minutes, until piping hot all the way through. Serve hot with your choice of vegetables alongside.

TO FREEZE: Leave until completely cooled, then cover the dish, either with a plastic lid or with a layer of clingfilm followed by a layer of foil, then label and transfer to the freezer for up to 3 months.

TO COOK FROM FROZEN: This can be defrosted overnight in the fridge or cooked directly from frozen. If defrosting first, cook as described left, until golden and bubbling. If cooking from frozen, increase the cooking time to 1 hour 10 minutes, covering with foil if the top starts to burn and ensuring a knife inserted into the centre is piping hot before serving.

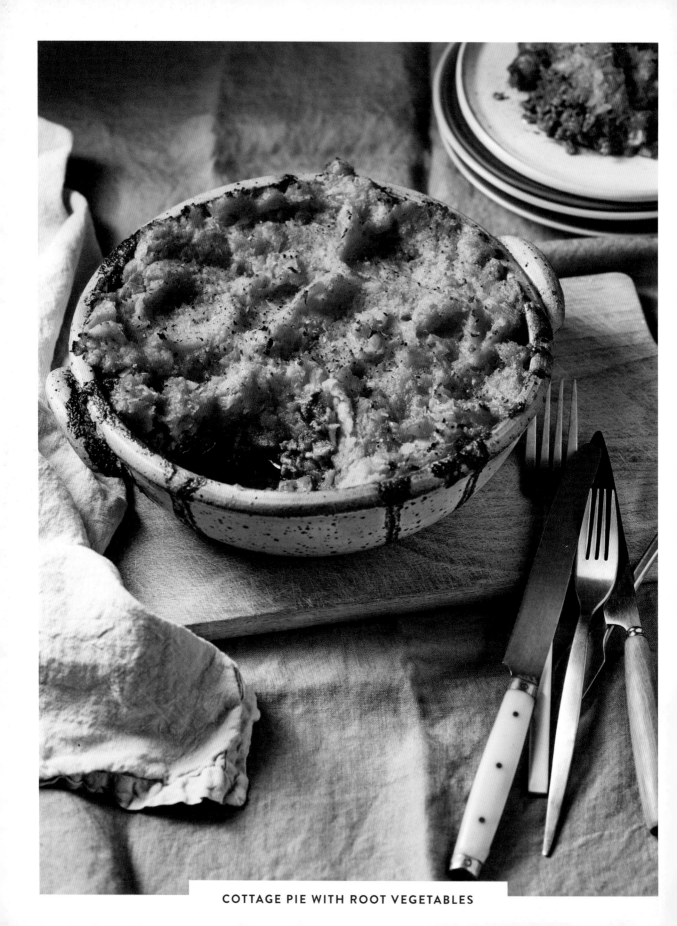

COTTAGE PIE WITH ROOT VEGETABLES

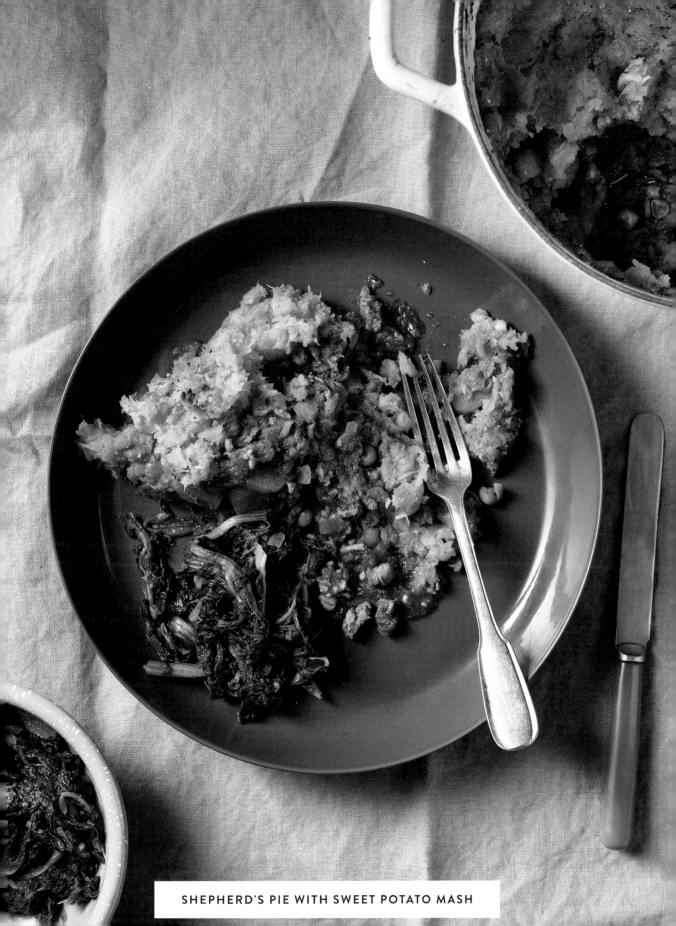

SHEPHERD'S PIE WITH SWEET POTATO MASH

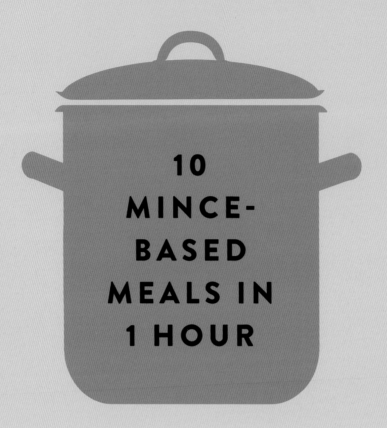

10 MINCE-BASED MEALS IN 1 HOUR

Are you ready to cook ten mince-based family meals in just 60 minutes? You will be making five recipes, each of which is doubled up to feed eight people, so just has to be split into two meals before freezing. The recipes are a mixture of cooked and no-cook meals, so while one recipe is bubbling away on the stove or cooking in the oven, you can be prepping the next for the freezer.

The shopping list on the opposite page includes everything you need and I've scaled up the ingredients so you know what size pack of each ingredient to buy. Once you have your shopping, lay the ingredients out in piles according to the groupings overleaf, so that you have exactly what you need for each recipe to hand. Then, simply follow the numbered guide and you can't go wrong!

Don't panic if this takes you more than an hour the first time you cook it – you will get quicker each time you make it. So, roll up your sleeves, get cooking and think about the time you'll be saving yourself in the future!

YOU WILL BE MAKING:

FAJITAS
BOLOGNESE SAUCE
CHILLI
BEEF BURGERS
MEATBALLS

SHOPPING LIST

Fresh

2 x 500g bags grated carrot

4.5kg lean, minced beef

1 carton eggs

Frozen

2 x 500g bags frozen, chopped onions

1 x 75g bag frozen, chopped garlic

1 x 500g bag frozen, sliced mushrooms

Storecupboard

6 x 400g tins chopped tomatoes

3 x 500g cartons passata

2 x 400g tins kidney beans

1 tube/tin tomato purée

1 small bottle American mustard

1 bottle Worcestershire sauce

1 jar dried rosemary or basil

4 tsp dried Italian herbs or oregano

3 tsp mild chilli powder

2 x 30g packs fajita seasoning

INGREDIENTS

GET ORGANIZED! Before you start make sure that your kitchen surfaces are cleared down, then lay all the ingredients out in individual piles according to the groupings on these two pages.

FAJITAS, BOLOGNESE SAUCE & CHILLI

For all 3 dishes:

splash of olive oil

6 cups (690g) frozen, chopped onions

3kg lean, minced beef

6 cups (810g) grated carrot

For the Fajitas:

2 x 30g packs fajita seasoning

2 cups (150g) frozen, sliced peppers (optional)

For the Bolognese Sauce and Chilli:

2 tsp frozen, chopped garlic

3 cups (210g) frozen, chopped mushrooms

6 x 400g tins chopped tomatoes

3 x 500g cartons passata

4 tsp dried Italian herbs or dried oregano

4 tbsp tomato purée

For the Chilli:

3 tsp mild chilli powder

2 x 400g cans kidney beans, drained and rinsed

BEEF BURGERS

750g lean, minced beef

3 tbsp American mustard

6 tbsp Worcestershire sauce

1 egg, beaten

MEATBALLS

750g lean, minced beef

8 tbsp Worcestershire sauce

2 tbsp dried rosemary or basil

1 egg, beaten

METHOD

FAJITAS, BOLOGNESE SAUCE & CHILLI

01 Heat a splash of olive oil in a large pan, then add the onions, minced beef and grated carrot, stirring to break up the mince. Leave to cook, stirring occasionally, for 10–15 minutes, until the mince has browned.

BEEF BURGERS

02 Put all the ingredients for the Burgers into a bowl and bring together with your hands, mixing until well combined.

03 Divide the mixture into quarters, then halve again, leaving you with eight equal-sized portions of meat. Roll each portion of meat into a ball with your hands, then press down to form a patty.

04 Transfer the Burgers to a labelled freezer bag and freeze flat for up to 3 months.

MEATBALLS

05 Stir the Fajita, Bolognese and Chilli meat mixture in the pot to prevent it from sticking, then put all the ingredients for the Meatballs into a bowl and bring together with your hands, mixing until well combined. (To save on washing up, use the same bowl for both the Burgers and the Meatballs.)

06 Divide the mixture into two even halves, then divide each half into eight equal-sized pieces. Finally, divide each piece of meat in half again, leaving you with 32 portions.

07 Roll each piece of meat into a ball shape with your hands, then divide the meatballs between two labelled freezer bags and freeze flat for up to 3 months.

08 Clean down the kitchen, putting away anything that was used to make the Burgers or Meatballs.

09 The meat in your pan should now be browned, so remove from the heat and drain off any fat.

10 To finish making the Fajita mixture, set two labelled freezer bags on the counter and scoop 2 cups of the cooked mince, onion and carrot mixture into each. Add one packet of the fajita seasoning to each bag and gently shake to combine, then set aside until cooled to room temperature while you finish making the Bolognese and Chilli recipes.

11 Return the pan with the cooked mince, onion and carrot mixture to the stove and add the garlic, mushrooms, chopped tomatoes, passata, oregano and tomato purée, then stir to combine and leave to cook for 10 minutes, until the sauce has thickened. While the sauce is cooking, clean down your kitchen.

12 To finish making the Bolognese sauce, set two labelled freezer bags on the counter and scoop 4 cups of the meat mixture into each bag. Set aside until cooled to room temperature while you finish making the Chilli recipe.

13 To finish making the Chilli, add the chilli powder and drained kidney beans to the remaining meat in the pan and stir to combine. Set two labelled freezer bags on the counter and divide the remaining meat mixture between them, there should be roughly enough for four cups in each bag.

14 Once the Fajita mix has cooled to room temperature, add a cup of sliced peppers to each bag, if using, and freeze flat for up to 3 months.

15 Once the bags of Bolognese Sauce and Chilli have cooled to room temperature, freeze flat for up to 3 months.

Congratulations!
You now have 10 evening meals ready for the freezer!

WHEN YOU COME TO COOK

Once cooked and frozen, all of these meals are best fully defrosted before cooking. All reheated meals should reach a temperature of 74°C/165°F. Always make sure any reheated food is piping hot before serving. Cooking times for each dish are listed below.

FAJITAS

Once defrosted, transfer to a heatproof bowl and cook on high in the microwave for 4 minutes, until piping hot. Alternatively, transfer to a pan and heat over a medium-high heat, stirring occasionally, until piping hot.

BOLOGNESE

Once defrosted, transfer to a heatproof bowl and cook on high in the microwave for 4 minutes, until piping hot. Alternatively, transfer to a pan and heat over a medium-high heat, stirring occasionally, until piping hot.

CHILLI

Once defrosted, transfer to a heatproof bowl and cook on high in the microwave for 4 minutes, until piping hot. Alternatively, transfer to a pan and heat over a medium-high heat, stirring occasionally, until piping hot.

BURGERS

Once defrosted, fry in a little oil for 2–3 minutes on each side. Alternatively, bake in an oven pre-heated to 200°C/400°F/gas mark 6 for 10–15 minutes, turning halfway through cooking.

MEATBALLS

Once defrosted, fry in a little oil for 5–6 minutes, turning the meatballs as you cook them. Alternatively, bake in an oven preheated to 200°C/400°F/gas mark 6 for 20 minutes, turning halfway through cooking.

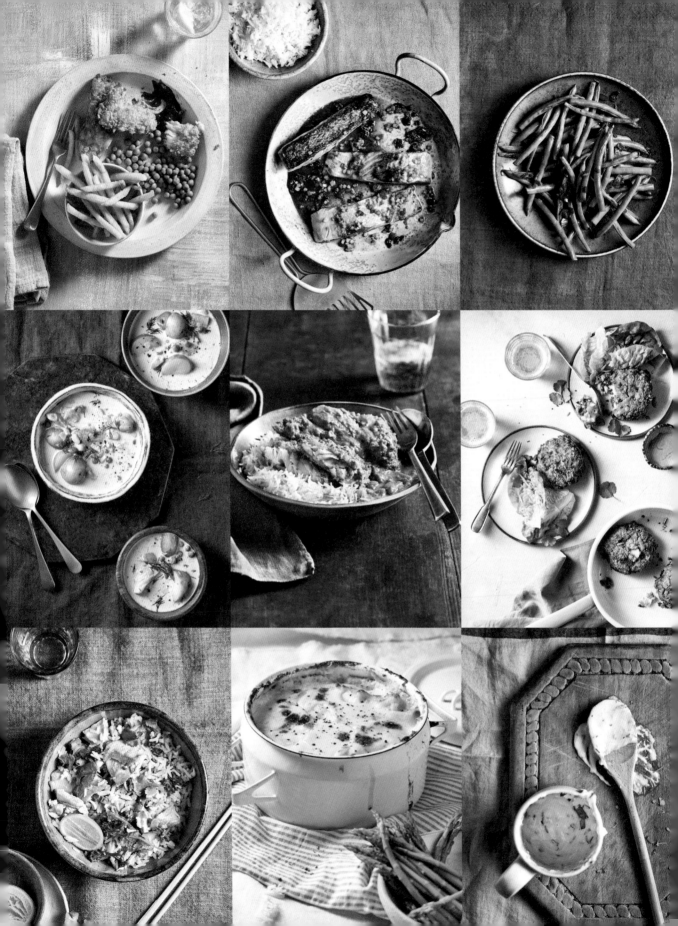

FISH

Light, fresh and healthy, my family love fish and I try and cook it at home at least twice a week. If you're new to cooking with fish, don't be intimidated – the recipes here are all very quick and simple to make and are perfect for batching.

The benefit of batching fish dishes is that they are often very quick to cook and, though some fish can be expensive, it is easily bulked out with vegetables, meaning that just a little bit goes a long way. The recipes in this chapter cover everything from family favourites, such as comforting fish pie and creamy chowder to more exotic fare, such as Katsu Fish Curry and Thai Sweet Potato Fish Cakes, meaning that you will find delicious meals for every night of the week!

LUXURY SEAFOOD CHOWDER

PREP: 10 MINUTES
COOK: 20 MINUTES
SERVES 4–6

splash of oil
1 cup (115g) frozen,
   chopped onions
1½ tbsp plain flour
4 cups (960ml) vegetable
   or fish stock
300g baby new potatoes,
   halved
1¼ cups (300ml) whole milk
½ cup (120ml) double cream
1 cup (140g) frozen
   sweetcorn
1 cup (155g) frozen peas
600g fresh fish pie mix
1 small pack fresh dill,
   leaves, finely chopped
   (optional), to serve
salt and freshly ground
   pepper

This hearty soup is packed with delicious chunks of fish and filling potatoes, making it a great winter warmer. For an extra flourish, why not serve it in a hollowed-out roll, just as they do in Boston.

01 Heat a splash of oil in a large pan over a high heat, then add the onions and cook for 1 minute, stirring continuously, until softened. Add the flour to the pan, stir to combine with the onions, then pour in the stock.

02 Add the potatoes to the pan and season to taste. Bring the stock to a boil, then reduce the heat to a simmer and leave to cook for 10–12 minutes, until the potatoes are just tender.

While the potatoes are cooking, make the Fish Pie.

03 Once the potatoes are cooked, add the remaining ingredients to the pan, stir to combine and leave to simmer for 5–6 minutes, until the fish has cooked through.

TO SERVE: Ladle the Chowder into serving bowls and serve hot, sprinkled with fresh dill and with fresh crusty bread or cheese scones alongside.

TO FREEZE: Leave the Chowder to cool completely, then ladle into a labelled, freezer or soup bag, removing as much air as possible from the bag as you seal it. Transfer to the freezer and freeze flat for up to 3 months.

TO COOK FROM FROZEN: Remove the Chowder from the freezer and allow to defrost completely in your fridge, then transfer to a pan over a medium heat until piping hot. Serve as described left.

EASY-BUT-LUXURY
FISH PIE

PREP: 5 MINUTES
COOK: 30 MINUTES
SERVES 4

400g fresh fish pie mix
1 cup (140g) frozen
  sweetcorn
1 cup (155g) frozen peas
1 small pack fresh dill,
  leaves finely chopped
1½ cups (360ml) double
  cream
425g (about 1½ packs)
  ready-made mashed
  potatoes

This pie takes just moments to put together and tastes amazing. If you are making this for the freezer, work as fast as you can to ensure the frozen veg in the pie does not thaw out between freezes.

01 Put the fish mix, sweetcorn and peas in the base of a large baking dish and sprinkle over the dill. Pour over the cream and give everything a stir to combine.
02 Spoon the mashed potatoes over the fish mixture, then spread over the top with a spatula or palette knife to form an even layer.

Zhuzh it Up!
To add even more luxury to both of these dishes, add some prawns or even lobster tails to the fish mix before cooking

TO COOK: Cook the pie on an oven preheated to 200°C/400°F/gas mark 6 for 30 minutes, until bubbling and golden.

TO FREEZE: Cover the pie with a lid, or wrap in a layer of clingfilm followed by a layer of foil, then label and freeze flat for up to 3 months.

TO COOK FROM FROZEN: This can be defrosted or cooked from frozen. If defrosted, cook as described left. If cooking from frozen, increase the cooking time to 1 hour, covering with foil if the top starts to catch.

FISH

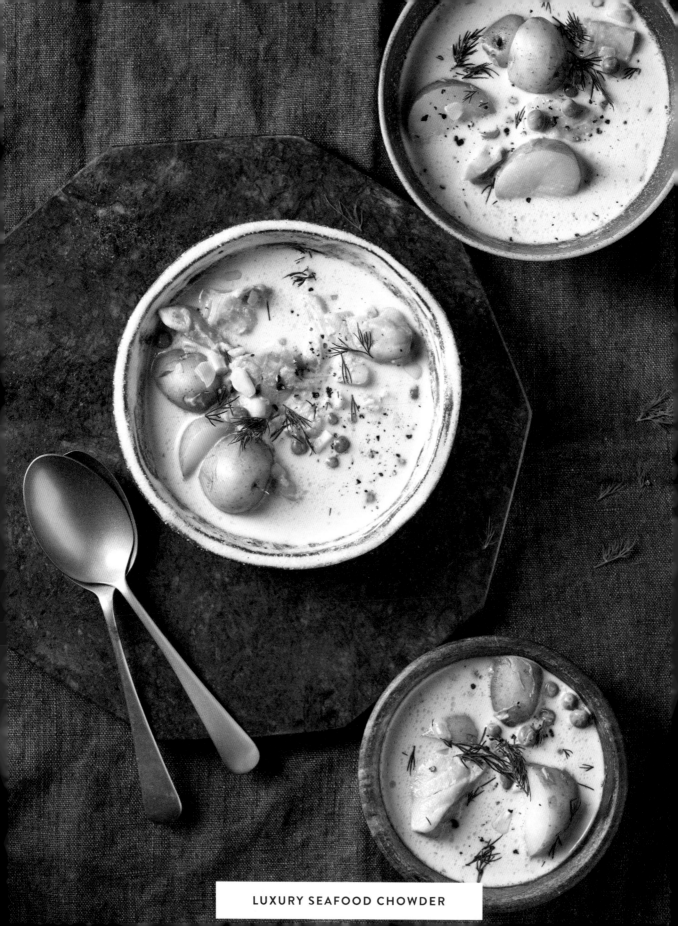

LUXURY SEAFOOD CHOWDER

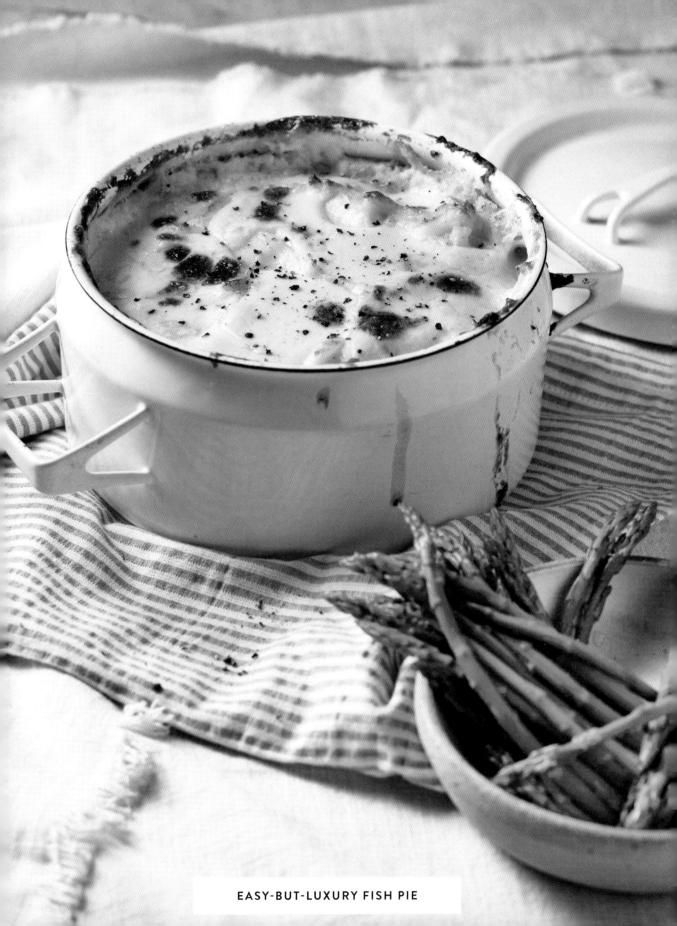

EASY-BUT-LUXURY FISH PIE

SALMON FRIED RICE

PREP: 15 MINUTES
COOK: 15 MINUTES

2 cups (360g) basmati rice
3 tbsp sesame or olive oil
2–3 salmon fillets
(100–150g each)
1 x 365g can sweetcorn,
drained
2 cups (300g) chopped,
frozen mixed vegetables
½ cup (120ml) soy sauce
3 eggs, beaten

This is a great one-pot meal that can be made fresh or frozen for later. If you don't eat fish, simply substitute it for more vegetables or meat of your choice.

01 Cook the rice in a pan of boiling water over a medium heat according to packet instructions. Once cooked, drain, rinse and set aside.

> While the rice is cooking, prepare the Chilli
> & Ginger Salmon Fillets, if you are making them to freeze.

02 Heat the oil in a frying pan over a medium heat, then add the salmon and cook for 3 minutes, removing and discarding the skin as the salmon cooks. Don't worry if the salmon flesh starts to break up as it cooks, this is necessary to distribute it through the rice in the finished dish.

03 Add the sweetcorn, frozen vegetables and soy sauce to the pan, then stir to combine. Using a wooden spoon or spatula, push the salmon and vegetable mixture to the side of the pan, then pour the beaten eggs into the centre and scramble them as they cook.

04 Add the rice to the pan, then stir everything until the salmon, vegetable and eggs are well distributed throughout the rice. Once the rice is piping hot, remove from the heat.

TO SERVE: The rice is now ready to be spooned into bowls and served warm.

TO FREEZE: Set the rice aside until cooled to room temperature, then spoon into a labelled freezer bag and freeze flat for up to 3 months. Alternatively, if you would like to cook the dish from frozen, spoon the cooled rice into a freezer-proof baking dish, cover with a layer of clingfilm followed by a layer of foil, label and freeze flat for up to 3 months.

TO COOK FROM FROZEN: The dish can be fully defrosted in the fridge or cooked from frozen. If defrosted, simply reheat the rice in a microwave or pan for 3–4 minutes, until piping hot. If cooking from frozen, remove the clingfilm and foil from the baking dish and cook in an oven preheated to 180°C/350°F/gas mark 4 for 30 minutes, until piping hot.

CHILLI & GINGER SALMON FILLETS

F

PREP: 5 MINUTES
COOK: 10 MINUTES
SERVES 4

4 salmon fillets (100–150g each)
6 tbsp dark soy sauce
1 tbsp chopped, frozen ginger
1 tbsp chopped, frozen red chilli
1 tsp chopped, frozen garlic
juice of 1 orange
To Serve:
splash of sesame or olive oil
cooked basmati rice

It takes just moments to pop all the ingredients for this healthy meal into a bag and put in the freezer. Then it can simply be whipped out of the freezer and defrosted when you want to serve it. What could be easier?

TO COOK: Heat the oil in a frying pan over a medium heat, then add the salmon and cook for 4 minutes on each side, until cooked through. Meanwhile, put the remaining ingredients in a small pan over a medium heat and stir to combine. Serve the cooked salmon fillets on a bed of rice with the hot sauce spooned over.

TO FREEZE: Put the soy sauce, ginger, chilli, garlic and orange juice into a labelled freezer bag and mix to combine, then add the salmon fillets, seal and freeze flat for up to 3 months.

TO COOK FROM FROZEN: Transfer the salmon bag to the fridge and allow to fully defrost, then remove the salmon from the bag and pan-fry in a splash of oil for 4 minutes on each side. Heat the sauce in a separate pan, then serve the dish as described in the *To Cook* section, left.

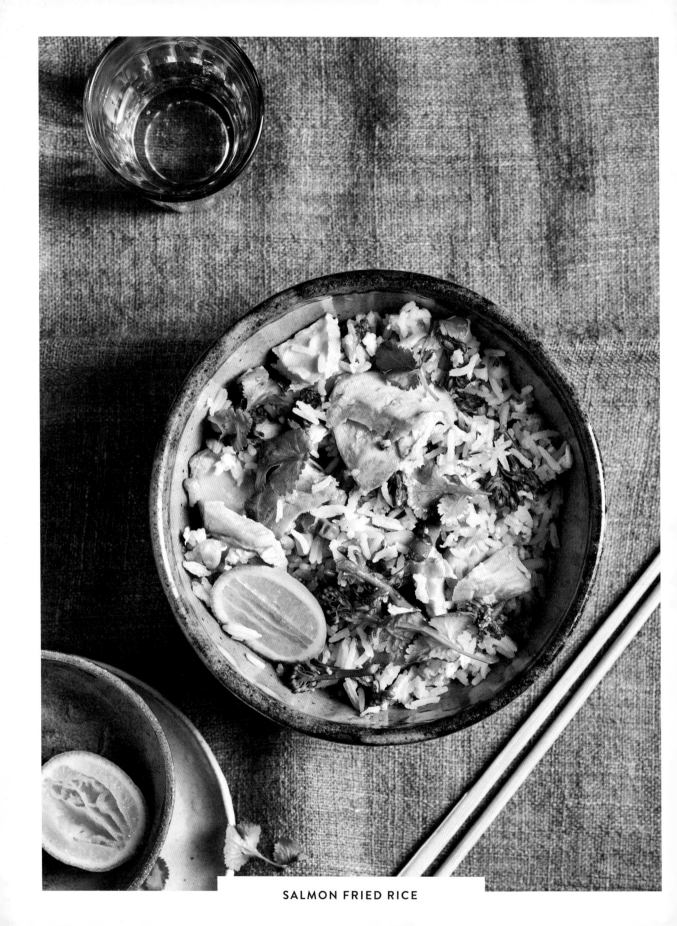

SALMON FRIED RICE

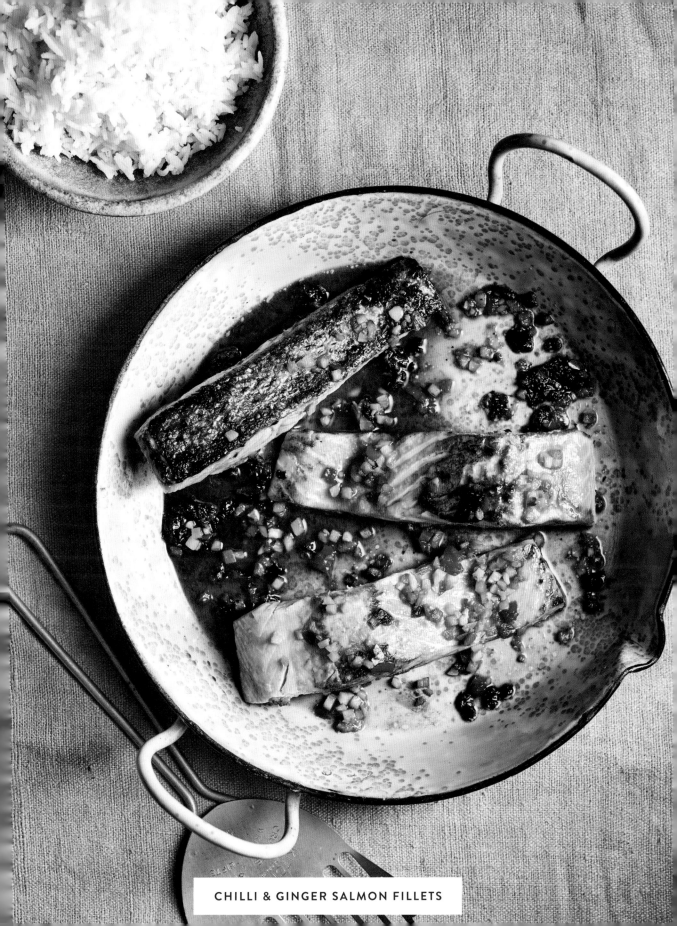

CHILLI & GINGER SALMON FILLETS

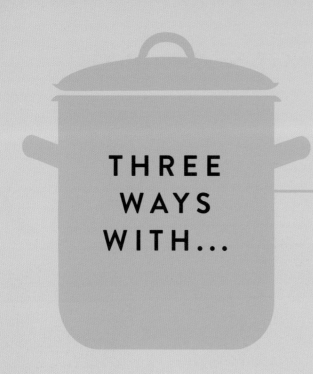

THREE WAYS WITH...

Now that you've prepared your Chilli & Ginger Salmon Fillets and have them stored in your freezer, what are you going to do with them? Below are three simple ideas for different ways of serving them that will keep mealtimes feeling fresh and different every time!

SALMON & CHILLI STIR-FRY

splash of sesame or vegetable oil
1 x quantity Chilli & Ginger
  Salmon Fillets (prepped as per
  the *To Freeze* instructions on
  page 127 and then defrosted)
4 nests dried noodles
1 x 300g pack mixed stir-fry
  vegetables
1 x 200g pack beansprouts
  (optional)

01 Heat a splash of oil in a large frying pan or wok over a medium heat, then remove the defrosted salmon fillets from the freezer bag and cook for 4 minutes on each side.

02 While the salmon is cooking, bring a pan of water to the boil, then add the noodles. Immediately remove the pan from the heat and set aside for 4 minutes to allow the noodles to cook.

03 Pour half of the liquid from the freezer bag into the pan with the salmon, then add the stir-fry vegetables and beansprouts, if using, and cook, stirring continuously, for 5 minutes. Don't worry if the salmon flesh starts to break up as you stir, this is necessary to distribute it through the finished dish.

04 Drain the noodles, then add them to the pan with the salmon and vegetables and stir to combine. Divide the mixture between four serving plates and serve hot.

LUXURY SALMON SALAD

splash of sesame or
   vegetable oil
1 x quantity Chilli & Ginger
   Salmon Fillets (prepped as per
   the *To Freeze* instructions on
   page 127 and then defrosted)
a large bowl of mixed salad
   of your choice – I like this
   to feel really generous, so
   add tomato, cucumber,
   watercress, sweetcorn and
   quartered boiled eggs to the
   salad leaves

01 Heat a splash of oil in a large frying pan over a
    medium heat, then remove the defrosted
    salmon fillets from the freezer bag and cook,
    skin-side down for 4 minutes.
02 Turn the salmon, then pour in the marinade
    from the freezer bag. Leave to cook for
    another 4 minutes, until the salmon is cooked
    through and the sauce has thickened to a
    sticky glaze.
03 Divide the salad between four serving plates,
    then top each with a salmon fillet. Spoon the
    sauce over to use as a dressing.

CHILLI & GINGER SALMON WITH STICKY RICE & SPRING ONIONS

splash of sesame or vegetable
   oil
1 x quantity Chilli & Ginger
   Salmon Fillets (prepped as per
   the *To Freeze* instructions on
   page 127 and then defrosted)
2 x 260g packs microwavable
   sticky rice
4 spring onions, sliced

01 Heat a splash of oil in a large frying pan over
    a medium heat, then remove the defrosted
    salmon fillets from the freezer bag and cook,
    skin-side down for 4 minutes.
02 Turn the salmon, then pour in the marinade
    from the freezer bag. Leave to cook for
    another 4 minutes, until the salmon is cooked
    through and the sauce has thickened to a
    sticky glaze.
03 While the salmon is cooking, cook the
    rice in the microwave according to packet
    instructions, then divide between 4 serving
    bowls. Spoon a salmon fillet onto each bed of
    rice and drizzle over the sauce. Scatter with
    sliced spring onions and serve hot.

F

THAI SWEET POTATO FISH CAKES

PREP: 10 MINUTES
COOK: 35 MINUTES
MAKES 8 PORTIONS

375g skinless, boneless cod fillet (fresh or frozen)
600g (1½ packs) ready-made sweet potato mash
1 cup (40g) chopped fresh coriander
3 spring onions, finely sliced
1 tbsp of soy sauce
2 cups (90g) panko breadcrumbs
2 eggs, beaten
splash of vegetable oil, for frying

01 Preheat the oven to 200°C/400°F/gas mark 6 and line a baking sheet with foil. Place the cod fillet on the prepared tray and transfer to the oven to cook for 15–20 minutes, until just cooked and starting to flake.

02 While the cod is cooking, put the sweet potato mash, coriander, spring onions and soy sauce in a large bowl and set aside. Put the panko breadcrumbs and beaten eggs in two separate shallow bowls and set them next to the bowl with the sweet potato mash.

While you are waiting for the cod to cook, make the Fish Goujons.

03 When the fish is cooked, flake it into the bowl with the sweet potato, then mix together until really well combined. Divide the mixture into eight equal-sized patties with your hands.

04 Dip the Fish Cakes in the beaten egg, then quickly in the panko breadcrumbs, ensuring they are well coated. Set aside and repeat until all of the fish cakes are ready to cook.

05 Heat a splash of oil in a frying pan over a medium-high heat, then cook the Fish Cakes in batches of four for 4 minutes on each side until crisp and golden.

TO SERVE: Serve the Fish Cakes warm with salad alongside.

TO FREEZE: Once cooled, transfer to a clearly labelled freezer bag in a single layer, then freeze flat for up to 3 months.

TO COOK FROM FROZEN: These can be defrosted or cooked directly from frozen. If defrosted, cook in an oven preheated to 180°C/350°F/gas mark 4 for 15 minutes. If cooking from frozen, increase the cooking time to 30 minutes.

PANKO FISH GOUJONS

PREP: 15 MINUTES
COOK: 5 MINUTES
SERVES 4

½ cup (65g) plain flour
2 cups (90g) panko
   breadcrumbs
small bunch of dill,
   chopped (optional)
2 eggs, beaten
vegetable oil, for frying
600g skinless, boneless
   cod fillet, cut into 2.5 x
   7cm (1 x 2¾in) pieces
salt and freshly ground
   pepper

01 Put the flour on a plate and season with salt and pepper. Put the panko breadcrumbs in a shallow bowl with the chopped dill (if using). Put the beaten eggs into a separate shallow bowl, then set all three dishes next to each other on the worktop.

02 Heat 1cm (½in) of vegetable oil in the base of a large frying pan over a medium-high heat.

03 While the oil is heating, dredge the pieces of cod in the flour, shaking off any excess, then dip in the egg, then roll in the panko breadcrumbs until coated. Set aside and repeat until all of the fish is coated.

04 Transfer the goujons to the hot oil and cook in batches, being careful not to overcrowd the pan, for 2 minutes, turning halfway through cooking. Transfer the cooked goujons to a plate lined with kitchen paper to remove any excess oil.

TO SERVE: The Goujons are now ready to serve. Kids love them with corn on the cob, peas and potato wedges alongside, but they would also be lovely inside a sandwich with lashings of mayo and ketchup.

TO FREEZE: Once the Goujons have cooled to room temperature, transfer to a labelled freezer bag and freeze flat for up to 1 month. I freeze these beside some corn, peas and frozen potato wedges, so that I have an entire meal ready to go.

TO COOK FROM FROZEN: Cook in an oven preheated to 180°C/350°F/gas mark 4 for 15–20 minutes, until piping hot.

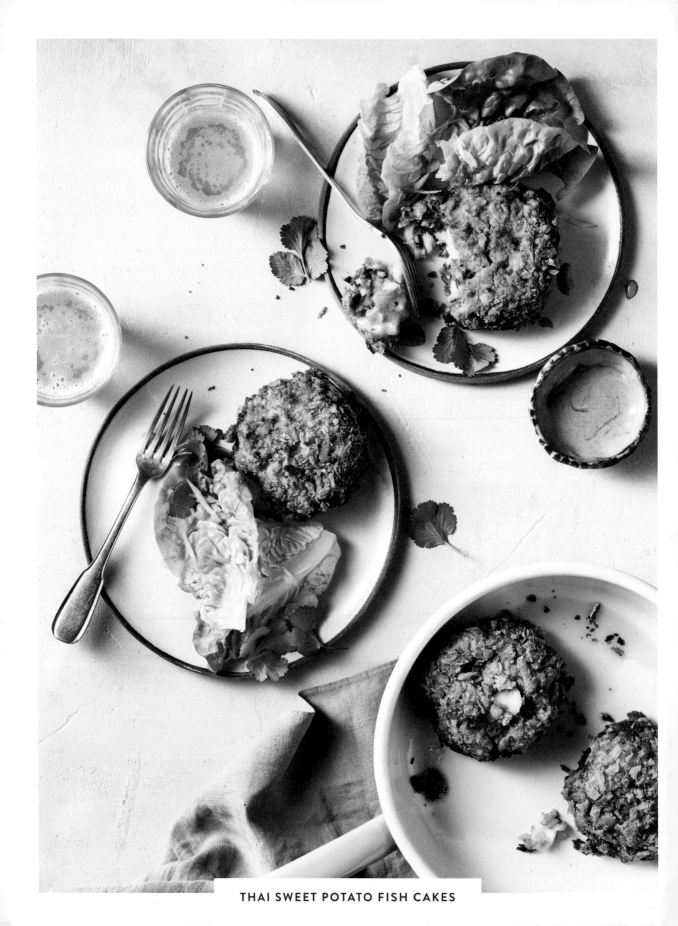

THAI SWEET POTATO FISH CAKES

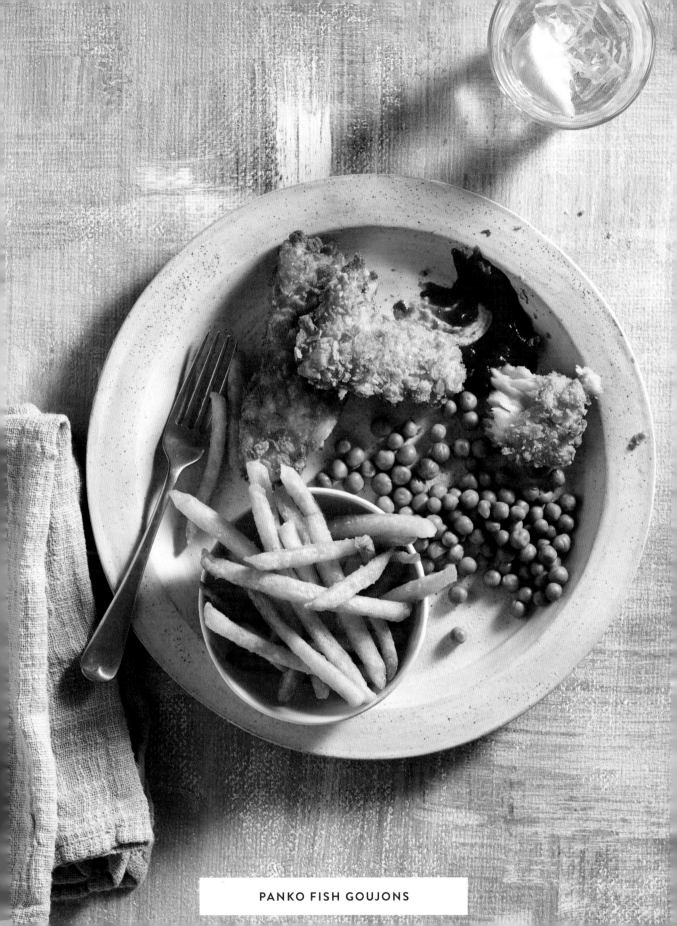

PANKO FISH GOUJONS

KATSU FISH CURRY

PREP: 15 MINUTES
COOK: 25 MINUTES
SERVES 4

2 cups (300g) frozen,
   chopped carrots
¾ cup (180ml) coconut
   milk
1 x 180g jar katsu curry
   paste
4 x panko-breaded, shop-
   bought cod fillets (if not
   breading your own)
cooked rice, to serve

If breading your own fish:
4 x skinless, boneless cod
   fillets (125–200g each)
1 cup (130g) plain flour
3 cups (130g) panko
   breadcrumbs
3 eggs, beaten
vegetable oil, for frying
salt and freshly ground
   pepper

This tasty, Japanese-inspired dish has lots of shortcuts that can make a simple dish even simpler! For speed, you can buy ready-breaded fish and microwave rice, meaning that all that's really left for you to do is make the sauce!

01 Bring a pan of water to the boil over a medium-high heat, add the carrots and cook for 5–7 minutes, then drain and set aside.

02 *If you are using fish fillets that are already breaded, skip the next 2 stages and continue from step 4.* While the carrots are cooking, put the flour on a plate and season generously with salt and pepper. Put the panko breadcrumbs in a shallow bowl, then put the beaten eggs in a separate shallow bowl. Set all 3 dishes next to each other on the worktop.

03 Dredge the fillets of cod in the flour, shaking off any excess, then dip in the egg and, finally, roll in the breadcrumbs until coated. Set aside and repeat until all of the fish is coated.

If you are also making the Chicken Katsu Burgers, clean down the breading station now and reset, then quickly bread the chicken.

04 Heat the coconut milk in a small pan over a low heat, then add the katsu paste, stir to combine and cook gently, stirring occasionally, until the mixture starts to simmer. Add the cooked carrots to the sauce, stir to combine, then remove the pan from the heat.

If you are also making the Chicken Katsu Burgers, hold back 1 tablespoon from the jar of the katsu paste to use when making them.

TO COOK: Transfer the fish to a baking sheet and cook in an oven preheated to 180°C/350°F/gas mark 5 for 15 minutes, until golden. Serve the fish on a bed of rice, with the warm katsu sauce spooned over.

TO FREEZE: Transfer the fish to a large, labelled freezer bag. Leave the sauce to cool to room temperature, then spoon into a smaller freezer bag, seal and place inside the bag with the fish. Freeze for up to 3 months.

TO COOK FROM FROZEN: This can be cooked from frozen. Cook the fish at 180°C/350°F/ gas mark for 20–25 minutes, until golden. Defrost the sauce in the microwave until piping hot, then serve as described in the *To Cook* section, left.

CHICKEN KATSU BURGERS (P)

PREP: 10 MINUTES
COOK: 15 MINUTES
SERVES 4

3 skinless, boneless chicken
   breasts
3–4 tbsp plain flour
1 tbsp mild curry powder
½ tsp salt
1 x 200g pack panko
   breadcrumbs
2 eggs, beaten
To Serve:
1 tbsp shop-bought katsu
   curry paste or 4 tbsp
   katsu curry sauce
4 tbsp mayonnaise (if using
   curry paste rather than
   sauce)
shredded lettuce and
   grated carrot
4 brioche burger buns,
   halved

This katsu curry/burger hybrid makes a great midweek meal and is a fun twist on the traditional way of serving chicken goujons. I like to serve these with corn on the cob alongside so, for ease, you could freeze a bag of corn alongside the goujons and pull it all out of the freezer at the same time.

01 Slice each of the chicken breasts into five long pieces, then set aside.
02 Put the flour, curry powder and salt on a plate and mix to combine. Put the panko breadcrumbs in a shallow bowl, then put the beaten eggs in a separate shallow bowl. Set all three dishes next to each other on the worktop.
03 Dredge the pieces of chicken in the flour, shaking off any excess, dip in the egg, then roll in the panko breadcrumbs until coated. Set aside and repeat until all of the chicken is coated.

Note
For a delicious meat-free version of these, substitute the chicken for sliced halloumi cheese and prepare in the same way.

TO COOK: Bake the chicken at 190°C/375°F/gas mark 5 for 10–15 minutes, until golden. If using the katsu paste, combine with the mayonnaise, then spread over the buns. Layer up the buns with the lettuce, carrot and a few of the goujons. If using katsu sauce, heat in a pan, and spoon the sauce over the chicken. Serve.

TO FREEZE: Transfer the coated chicken to a lined baking sheet, then transfer to the freezer for 3–4 hours. After this time, transfer to a labelled freezer bag and freeze flat for up to 1 month.

TO COOK FROM FROZEN: These can be cooked from frozen. Bake the chicken at 190°C/375°F/gas mark 5 for 15–20 minutes, until golden brown and the chicken is tender and juicy. Once cooked, assemble the burgers as described in the *To Cook* section, left.

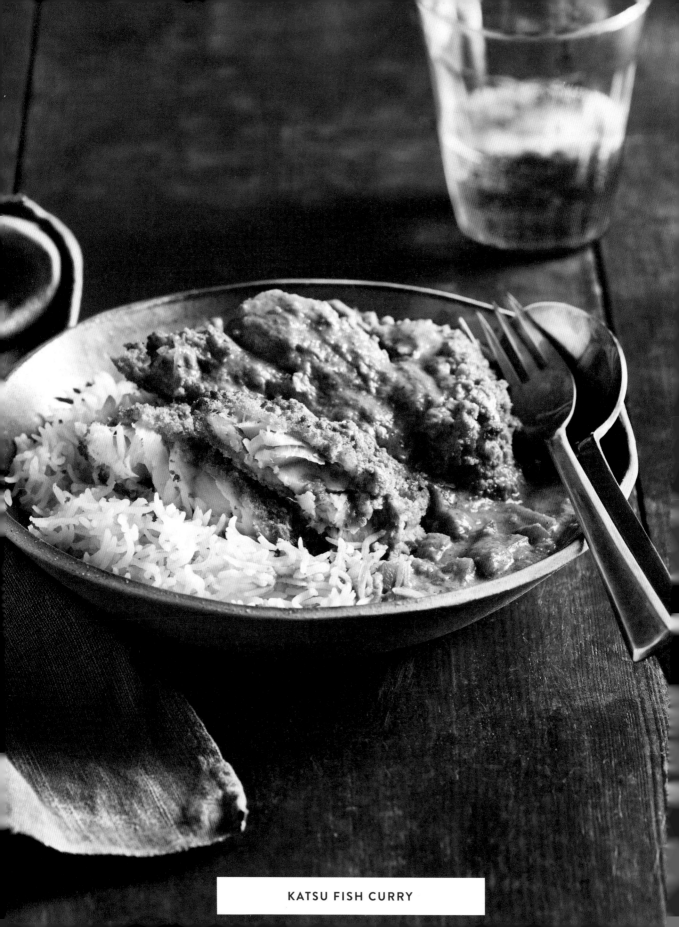

KATSU FISH CURRY

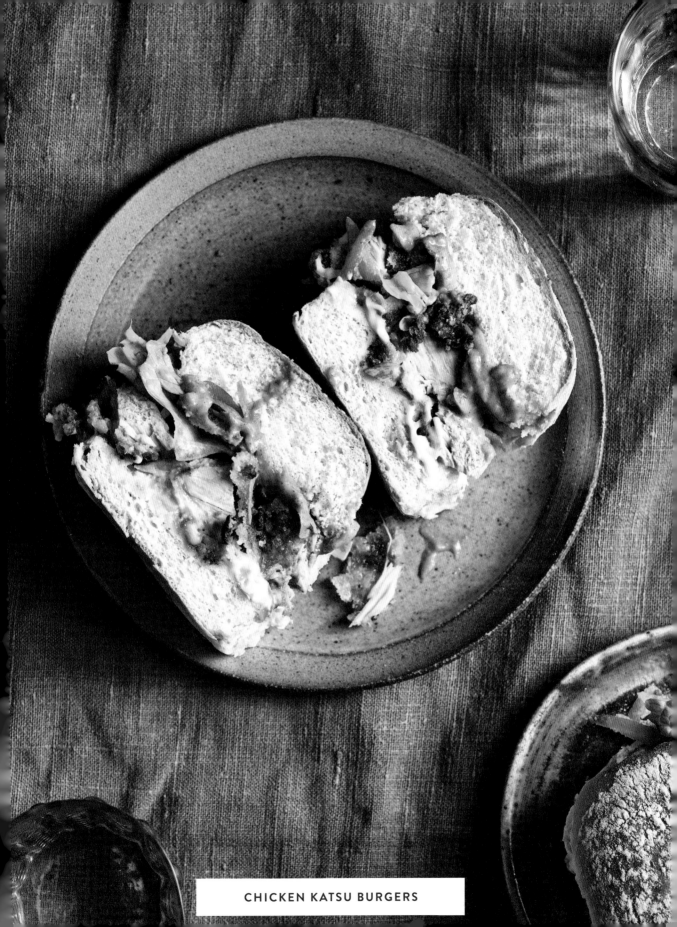

CHICKEN KATSU BURGERS

10
FISH
MEALS IN
1 HOUR

Are you ready to cook ten fish-based family meals in just 60 minutes? This method includes some of my favourite fish dishes, such as fish pie, fish chowder and panko goujons, which you can also find as individual recipes elsewhere in this chapter, though here they are scaled up to make a double portion and the methods are weaved together to make the best use of time. The recipes are a mixture of cooked and no-cook meals, so while one recipe is bubbling away, you can be prepping the next for the freezer.

The shopping list on the opposite page includes everything you need and I've scaled up the ingredients so you know what size pack to buy of each. Lay the ingredients out in piles according to the groupings overleaf, then follow the numbered guide and you can't go wrong!

Don't panic if this takes you more than an hour the first time you cook it – you will get quicker each time you make it. So, roll up your sleeves, get cooking and think about the time you'll be saving yourself in the future!

YOU WILL BE MAKING:

LUXURY FISH CHOWDER
LUXURY FISH PIE
CHILLI & GINGER SALMON FILLETS
LEMON & HERB COD PARCELS
PANKO FISH GOUJONS

SHOPPING LIST

Fresh

1 kg new potatoes

3 x 425g packs ready-made mashed potato

1 x 400g pack samphire

1 lemon

2 oranges

3 bunches fresh dill

6 x 400g packs fresh fish pie mix

2kg cod fillet

1.6kg cod loin

8 salmon fillets

16 rashers of smoked bacon

1 litre whole milk

2 x 600ml pot double cream

1 x 250g block unsalted butter

6 eggs

Frozen

1 x 500g bag frozen, chopped onions

1 x 700g pack frozen sweetcorn

1 x 700g pack frozen peas

1 x 75g pack frozen, chopped garlic

1 x 75g pack frozen, chopped ginger

1 x 75g pack frozen, chopped red chillies

Storecupboard

1 bottle olive or vegetable oil

1 pack fish stock cubes or 2 litres ready-made stock

1 bottle dark soy sauce

1 x 75g tube garlic purée

1 jar dried dill

1 x 500g bag plain flour

1 x 540g pack panko breadcrumbs

INGREDIENTS

LUXURY FISH CHOWDER

3 tbsp olive oil
2 cups (230g) frozen, chopped onions
3 tablespoons flour
8 cups (2 litres) fish or vegetable stock
1kg new potatoes, cut into cubes
2 cups (480ml) whole milk
1 cup (240 ml) double cream
4 x 400g packs fresh fish pie mix
2 cups (350g) frozen sweetcorn
2 cups (300g) of frozen peas
30g fresh chopped dill
salt and freshly ground pepper

LUXURY FISH PIE

2 x 400g packs fresh fish pie mix
2 cups (350g) frozen sweetcorn
2 cups (300g) frozen peas
60g fresh chopped dill
3 cups (720ml) double cream
3 x 425g packs ready-made mashed potatoes

CHILLI & GINGER SALMON FILLETS

12 tbsp dark soy sauce
2 tbsp frozen, chopped ginger
2 tbsp frozen, chopped red chillies
2 tsp frozen, chopped garlic
juice of 2 oranges
8 salmon fillets

LEMON & HERB COD LOIN

12 tbsp (170g) soft butter
3 tsp lemon juice
2 tsp garlic purée
3 tsp dried dill
4 skinless, boneless cod loins
  (approx. 300–400g each)
16 rashers of smoked back bacon
4 cups (400g) samphire

PANKO FISH GOUJONS

2 cups (260g) plain flour
6 cups (270g) panko breadcrumbs
60g fresh chopped dill
4–5 large eggs, beaten
vegetable oil, for frying
2kg skinless, boneless cod fillet, cut into 2.5 x
  7cm (1 x 2¾in) pieces
salt and freshly ground pepper

METHOD

LUXURY FISH CHOWDER

01 Heat a splash of oil in a large pan over a high heat, then add the onions and cook for 1 minute, stirring constantly, until softened. Add the flour to the pan, stir to combine with the onions, then pour in the stock.

02 Add the potatoes to the pan and season to taste. Bring the stock to a boil, then reduce the heat to a simmer and leave to cook for 10–12 minutes.

LUXURY FISH PIE

03 Divide the fish pie mix, sweetcorn and peas between the bases of two freezer-proof baking dishes and sprinkle over the dill. Pour half of the cream into each dish and give everything a stir to combine.

04 Crumble the mashed potatoes over the top of the two pies, then smooth over the top with a spatula or palette knife to form an even layer. Cover each pie with a lid or wrap in a layer of clingfilm followed by a layer of foil, label and freeze flat for up to 3 months.

LUXURY FISH CHOWDER CONTINUED...

05 Once the potatoes are tender, add the milk, cream, fish pie mix, sweetcorn, peas and dill to the pan and stir to combine. Leave to cook, stirring occasionally, for 10 minutes, then remove from the heat and set aside to cool.

CHILLI & GINGER SALMON FILLETS

06 Divide the soy sauce, ginger, chilli, garlic and orange juice between two large, labelled freezer bags and mix to combine, then add four salmon fillets to each bag, seal and freeze flat for up to 3 months.

PANKO FISH GOUJONS

07 Put the flour on a plate and season with salt and pepper. Put the panko breadcrumbs in a shallow bowl with the chopped dill (if using). Put the beaten eggs into a separate shallow bowl, then set all three dishes next to each other on the worktop.

08 Heat 1cm (½in) of vegetable oil in the base of a large frying pan over a medium-high heat.

09 While the oil is heating, dredge the pieces of cod in the flour, shaking off any excess, dip in the egg, then roll in the panko breadcrumbs until coated. Set aside and repeat until all of the fish is coated.

10 Transfer the Goujons to the hot oil and cook in batches, being careful not to overcrowd the pan, for 2 minutes, turning halfway through cooking. Transfer the cooked goujons to a plate lined with kitchen paper to remove any excess oil. Set aside to cool while you make the Lemon & Herb Cod Loin.

LEMON & HERB COD LOIN

11 Put the butter, lemon juice, garlic purée and dried dill in a small bowl and stir to combine.

12 Cut each cod loin in half widthways, then spread the butter mixture over the pieces of cod. Wrap each piece of buttered cod in two rashers of bacon.

13 Cut eight square pieces of foil, large enough to form a parcel around each piece of cod and set on your work surface. Divide the samphire between the squares of foil, piling it in the centre of each, then top each with one of the wrapped cod loins. Fold over each sheet of foil and crimp the edges together to form eight parcels. Transfer the parcels to 2 large, labelled freezer bags, seal and freeze flat for up to 3 months.

PANKO FISH GOUJONS CONTINUED...

14 Divide the cooled Goujons between 2 large labelled freezer bags and freeze flat for up to 3 months.

LUXURY FISH CHOWDER CONTINUED...

15 Once cooled to room temperature, divide the Chowder mixture between two large, labelled freezer bags, seal and freeze flat for up to 3 months.

Congratulations!
You now have 10 evening meals ready for the freezer!

WHEN YOU COME TO COOK

Once cooked and frozen, all of these meals are best fully defrosted before cooking. All reheated meals should reach a temperature of 74°C/165°F. Always make sure any reheated food is piping hot before serving. Cooking times for each dish are listed below.

LUXURY FISH CHOWDER

Once defrosted, transfer to a large pan and heat on the stovetop for 15 minutes, until piping hot.

LUXURY FISH PIE

Once defrosted, transfer to an oven preheated to 180°C/350°F/gas mark 4 for 30 minutes, until golden and bubbling.

CHILLI & GINGER SALMON FILLETS

Once defrosted, pan-fry the salmon in a little oil for 4 minutes each side, or until cooked through. Heat the sauce separately in the microwave or on the stove.

LEMON & HERB COD LOIN

Once defrosted, transfer the parcels to an oven preheated to 200°C/400°F/gas mark 6 for 20 minutes, opening the foil parcels for the last 10 minutes of cooking.

PANKO FISH GOUJONS

Once defrosted, transfer to an oven preheated to 180°C/350°F/gas mark 4 for 15–20 minutes, until golden.

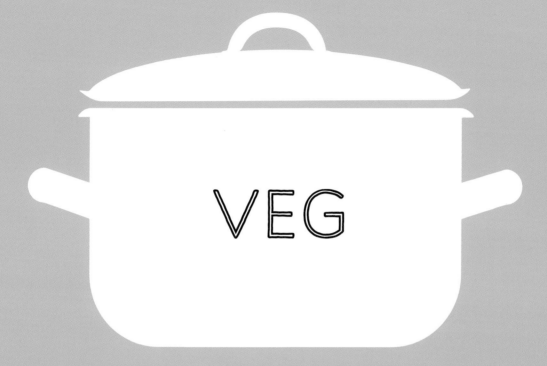

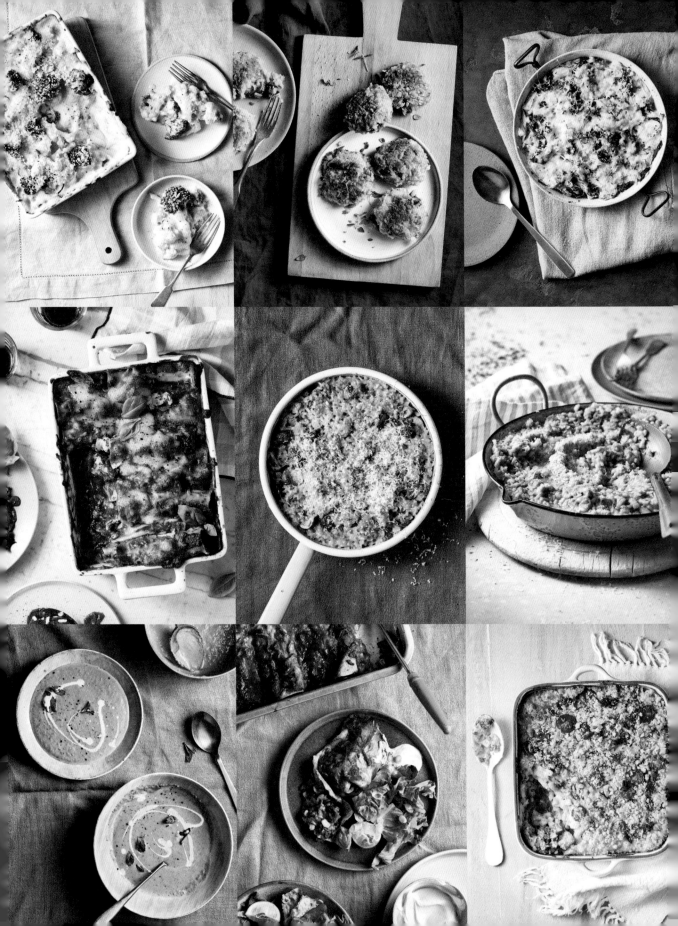

VEG

Whether for environmental, health or financial reasons, more and more of us are trying to reduce the amount of meat that we eat, whether that means cutting it out altogether, or just going meat-free a couple of times a week.

I live on a farm and until recently the meals that populated my weekly meal planner were predominantly meat based. Recently though, I have made a concerted effort to try to cook and serve a meat-free meal at least once a week and myself and my family have all loved the change.

The meals in this chapter are those that my family now love to eat. Not only will you find options for pasta, risotto and soup, I have also included many classic family favourites such as meat-free chilli and stuffed peppers. My favourite recipe in this chapter has to be the classic Scottish dish of Rumbledethumps (p.164). My husband and I love it so much that it was served as a late-night snack at our wedding – comfort food at its best!

VEGGIE BOLOGNESE

V

PREP: 10 MINUTES
COOK: 35 MINUTES
SERVES 4

2 cups (100g) store-
bought, pre-chopped
root vegetables (carrots,
parsnips and swede work
well)
1 cup (115g) frozen,
chopped onions
2 tsp frozen, chopped garlic
2 x 400g cans chopped
tomatoes
1 x 500g carton passata
2 tsp dried oregano
½ cup (100g) red lentils,
rinsed
1 cup (70g) chopped
mushrooms
cooked pasta or jacket
potatoes, to serve
grated cheese, to serve

Whether you are vegetarian, cutting down on meat or just looking to sneak a few extra vegetables into your kids, this is a great recipe. It's also easy, healthy and low calorie, making it the perfect midweek meal.

01 Cook the chopped root vegetables in a microwave for 10 minutes, until just tender. Alternatively, cook the vegetables in a pan of boiling water over a medium heat.

02 While the vegetables are cooking, heat a splash of oil in a large pan over a medium heat, then add the onions and garlic and cook, stirring, for 1 minute, until the onions have softened.

03 Add the chopped tomatoes, passata, oregano and lentils to the pan and stir to combine. Once the root vegetables have finished cooking, add those to the pan, too, then simmer for 20 minutes, remembering to stir occasionally, until the lentils are tender.

If you are also making the Chilli Bean Burgers, do so now while the Bolognese is simmering.

TO COOK: Add the mushrooms to the pan and stir to combine, then leave to cook for 5 minutes until the mushrooms are tender. Serve hot, spooned over cooked pasta or jacket potatoes and dredged in grated cheese.

TO FREEZE: Set aside to cool to room temperature, then scoop the mixture into a large, labelled freezer bag. Add the raw chopped mushrooms to the bag, then seal flat and transfer to the freezer for up to 3 months.

TO COOK FROM FROZEN: Defrost in the fridge, then cook in a large pan over a medium heat until piping hot and the mushrooms are cooked through. Alternatively, cook in the microwave for 10 minutes, stirring halfway through.

CHILLI BEAN BURGERS

V

PREP: 5 MINUTES
COOK: 8 MINUTES
SERVES 4

1 x 400g can three bean
 salad
120g (½ can) kidney beans
 (drained weight)
1 cup (40g) dried
 breadcrumbs
½ cup (70g) tinned
 sweetcorn (drained
 weight)
1 egg, beaten
1½ tsp chilli powder
1 small bunch coriander,
 leaves chopped
4 brioche buns (optional)
To Serve:
splash of olive oil (if pan
 frying)
store-bought salsa and
 guacamole
shredded lettuce leaves

Friday night is burger night in our house, and this delicately spiced, meat-free version is packed with flavour. Served in fluffy brioche buns and dressed with salsa, guacamole and fresh salad, this is a delicious meal that can be cooked straight from frozen, making it so easy to pop in the oven as soon you walk through the door.

01 Put both types of beans in a large bowl with the breadcrumbs, sweetcorn, beaten egg, chilli powder and coriander, then mix everything together with your hands until well combined.

02 Divide the mixture into four equal-sized balls, then flatten each ball into a patty, roughly the size of a burger bun.

TO COOK: Heat a splash of olive oil in a frying pan, then cook the burgers for 4 minutes on each side, until golden. Dress the buns with guacamole and salsa, top with the Bean Burgers and place some of the lettuce on top. Place the other halves of the burger buns on top and serve.

TO FREEZE: Transfer the burgers to a labelled freezer bag, then place the bag on a baking sheet and freeze flat for up to 3 months. Freeze a bag of buns, frozen potato wedges or corn on the cob alongside, for a full meal that's easy to grab from the freezer.

TO COOK FROM FROZEN: These can be defrosted or cooked from frozen. If defrosted, cook and assemble the burgers as described left. If frozen, cook in an oven preheated to 200°C/400°F/gas mark 6 for 25–30 minutes, until piping hot all the way through.

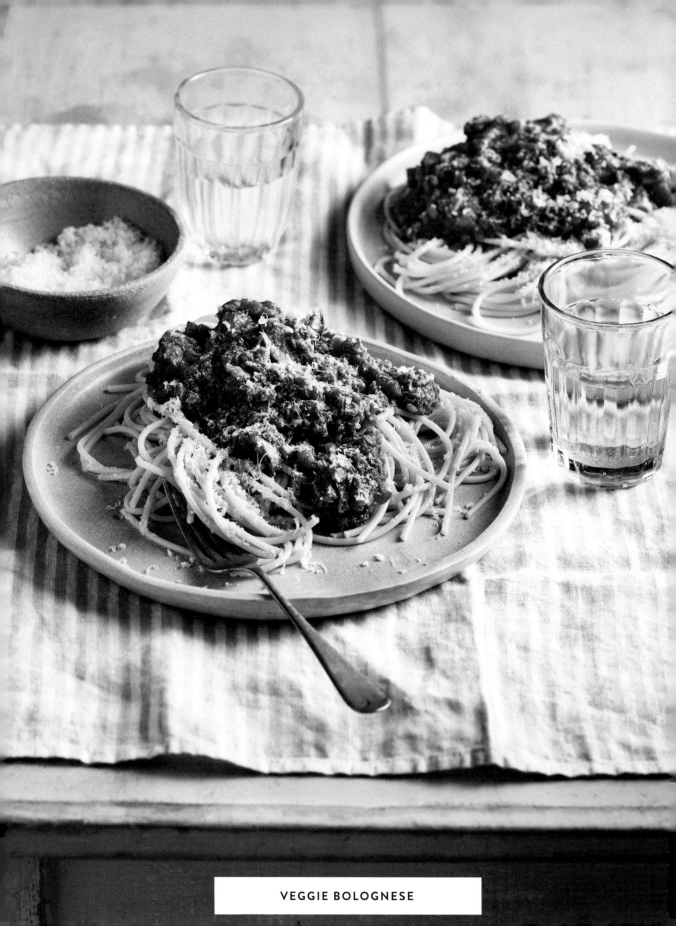

VEGGIE BOLOGNESE

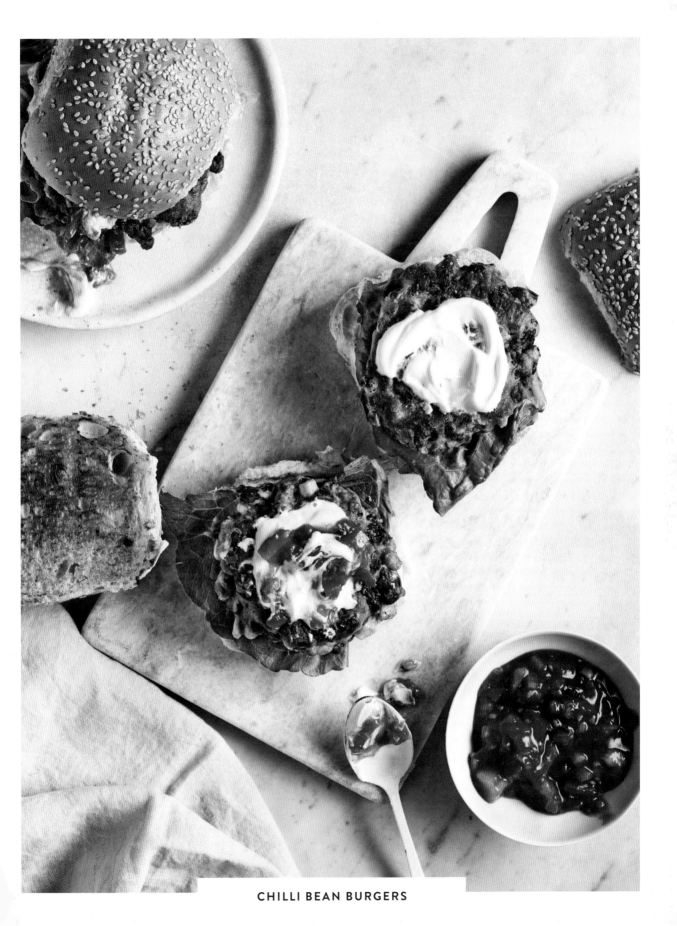

CHILLI BEAN BURGERS

BROCCOLI & CAULIFLOWER CHEESE BAKE

PREP: 15 MINUTES
COOK: 20 MINUTES
SERVES 4

1 cauliflower, cut into
   florets
1 broccoli, cut into florets
1 x quantity Cheese Sauce
   (p.207)
½ cup (60g) grated
   cheese, to serve
½ cup (55g) dried
   breadcrumbs, to serve

If you have some Cheese Sauce in the freezer ready to go, this can be assembled in moments. It makes a lovely side dish to roast meats, but is also a wonderfully comforting main course in its own right.

01 Heat a large pan of water over a high heat until boiling, then add the cauliflower and broccoli and cook for 5–6 minutes, until just tender but still retaining some bite.

If you don't have a batch of Cheese Sauce (p.207) ready to go, make it now while the cauliflower and broccoli are cooking. If you are also making the Luxury Macaroni Cheese Bake, simply double the recipe for the Cheese Sauce and put the macaroni onto boil at the same time as the cauliflower and broccoli.

02 Drain the cauliflower and broccoli through a colander, then tip the vegetables into the base of a large baking dish. Pour over the cheese sauce, then stir gently to make sure that the vegetables are well coated in the sauce.

TO COOK: Scatter the grated cheese and breadcrumbs over the top, then transfer to an oven preheated to 180°C/350°F/gas mark 4 for 15–20 minutes, until the top is golden and the sauce is bubbling. Serve hot.

TO FREEZE: Leave to cool to room temperature, then cover with a lid or a layer of clingfilm followed by a layer of foil. Clearly label the dish, then freeze flat for up to 3 months.

TO COOK FROM FROZEN: This can be cooked from frozen. Cover with foil, then cook in an oven preheated to 180°C/350°F/gas mark 4 for 1 hour, removing the foil and scattering over the cheese and breadcrumbs for the last 15 minutes.

LUXURY MACARONI CHEESE BAKE

M

PREP: 20 MINUTES
COOK: 20 MINUTES
SERVES 4

2 cups (240g) dried
  macaroni
1 x quantity Cheese Sauce
  (p.207)
1 cup (150g) cubed, cooked
  ham (omit if vegetarian)
16 cherry tomatoes, halved
½ cup (60g) grated
  cheese, to serve
½ cup (55g) dried
  breadcrumbs, to serve

This is a great recipe for when you have some Cheese Sauce (p.207) ready to go in the freezer. This version is packed with ham and tomatoes and topped with golden breadcrumbs for a luxurious finish but, for speed, you can omit the topping and the extra filling ingredients and serve the pasta stirred through the cheesy sauce. Either way, it's pure comfort food.

01 Bring a large pan of salted, boiling water to the boil over a high heat, then add the pasta and cook for 8–10 minutes, until tender but still retaining some bite.

If you don't have a batch of Cheese Sauce (p.207) ready to go, make it now while the pasta is cooking.

02 Drain and rinse the pasta through a colander, then add to a pan with the cheese sauce. Stir to combine, then add the cubed ham and halved cherry tomatoes and stir again. Pour the mixture into a large baking dish.

Zhuzh it Up!
To give this a more grown-up twist, add some chopped garlic and fresh, chopped parsley to the cheese sauce.

TO COOK: Scatter the grated cheese and breadcrumbs over the top, then transfer to an oven preheated to 180°C/350°F/gas mark 4 for 15–20 minutes, until the top is golden and the sauce is bubbling. Serve hot.

TO FREEZE: Leave to cool to room temperature, then cover with a lid or a layer of clingfilm followed by a layer of foil. Clearly label the dish, then freeze flat for up to 3 months.

TO COOK FROM FROZEN: This can be cooked from frozen. Cover with foil, then cook in an oven preheated to 180°C/350°F/gas mark 4 for 1 hour, removing the foil and scattering over the cheese and breadcrumbs for the last 15 minutes.

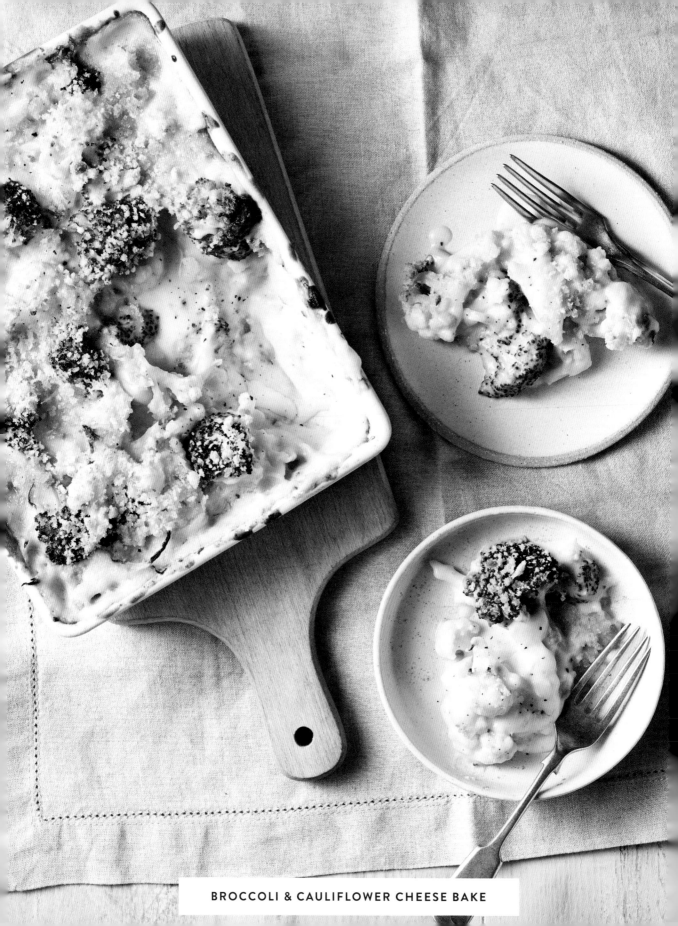

BROCCOLI & CAULIFLOWER CHEESE BAKE

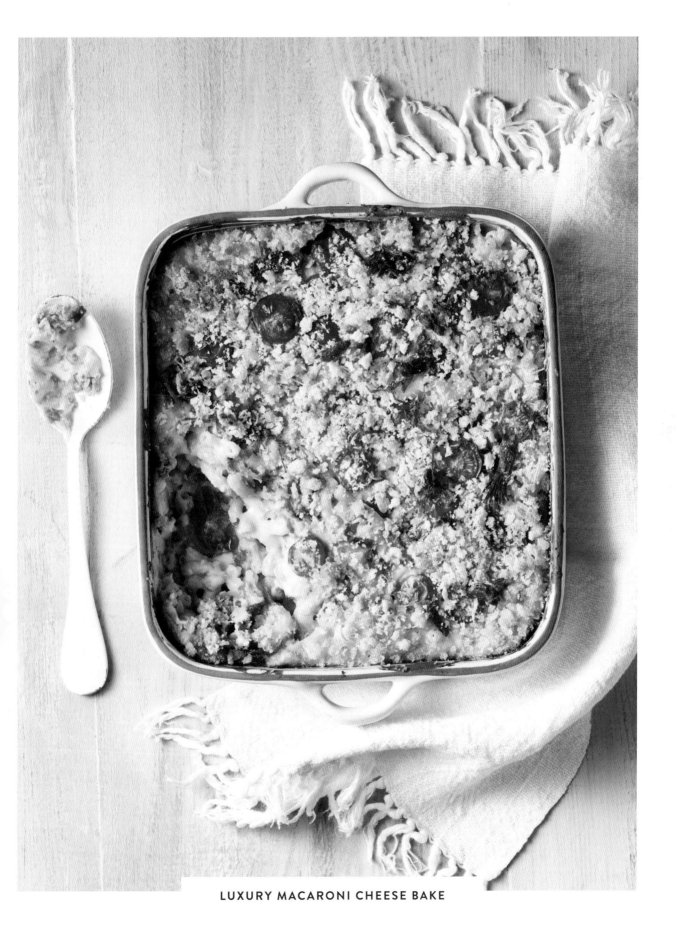

LUXURY MACARONI CHEESE BAKE

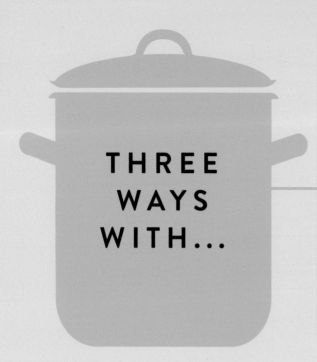

THREE WAYS WITH...

MACARONI CHEESE

Macaroni cheese is the ultimate comfort food, no matter what age you are. For a grown-up twist try adding some luxurious lobster tail to the mix, as below, or, if you are catering for a younger audience, the two variations on the opposite page are perfect for babies and young children.

MACARONI CHEESE LOBSTER POTS

1 x quantity Luxury Macaroni and Cheese Bake (p.154, made to the end of step 2)

2 tbsp butter

1 tsp frozen, chopped garlic

2 lobster tails, halved down the middle

½ cup (55g) breadcrumbs

1 cup (115g) grated gruyere cheese

01 Preheat the oven to 180°C/350°F/gas mark 4, then divide the Luxury Macaroni Cheese Bake between four ramekins and set aside.

02 Melt the butter and garlic in a frying pan over a medium heat, then add the halved lobster tails and cook for 5 minutes, turning and coating with the butter and garlic mixture occasionally.

03 Add half a lobster tail to each ramekin and stir to incorporate into the Macaroni Cheese, then scatter breadcrumbs and gruyere cheese over the top of each. Transfer to the oven and cook for 15 minutes, until golden. Serve hot.

MACARONI CHEESE FOR TODDLERS & SMALL CHILDREN

2 cups (240g) small dried
macaroni
1 x quantity Cheese Sauce (see
page 207), made omitting the
Dijon mustard
1 cup (150g) cubed, cooked
ham
½ cup (60g) grated cheese, to
serve
½ cup (55g) dried breadcrumbs,
to serve

01 Make the Luxury Macaroni Cheese Bake to
the end of step 2, omitting the tomatoes and
the mustard from the cheese sauce and using
the smallest dried macaroni you can find.

02 Divide the mixture into individual
ramekins for easy portioning, then top
with breadcrumbs and cheese and freeze
or bake as per the original recipe.

MACARONI CHEESE BABY FOOD

2 cups (240g) small dried
macaroni
1 x quantity Cheese Sauce (see
page 207), made omitting the
Dijon mustard
1 cup (150g) cubed, cooked
ham
splash of milk

01 Make the Luxury Macaroni Cheese Bake to
the end of step 2, omitting the tomatoes and
the mustard from the cheese sauce and using
the smallest dried macaroni you can find.

02 Using a blender or hand blender, process the
macaroni cheese until smooth, adding a splash
of milk if the mixture is too thick. Spoon
the mixture into silicone ice cube trays
and leave to cool, then freeze flat for up to
3 months, removing and defrosting individual
cubes as needed.

SPINACH & RICOTTA CANNELLONI

PREP: 20 MINS
COOK: 40 MINS
SERVES 6

8 cubes frozen, chopped
   spinach
2 x 250g tubs ricotta
   cheese
1 tsp ground nutmeg
1 x quantity Basic Tomato
   Sauce (see page 200) or
   1 large jar store-bought
   tomato sauce
12 dried cannelloni shells
1 cup (115g) grated
   mozzarella cheese
   (optional)

01 Put the frozen spinach in a heatproof bowl and cook in the microwave on high for 2½ minutes, then stir and cook for 2 minutes more. Drain the spinach through a colander lined with kitchen paper, pressing down to remove as much liquid as possible, then return the spinach to the bowl.

If you are also making the Stuffed Chicken recipe, cook the spinach for both recipes together, then divide into separate bowls before adding the ricotta for each recipe.

02 Add the ricotta cheese and nutmeg to the bowl with the spinach, stir to combine and set aside. Pour half of the tomato sauce into the base of a large baking dish.

03 Using your hands or a teaspoon, fill the cannelloni shells with the spinach and ricotta mixture, then lay them in an even layer over the tomato sauce in the base of the baking dish.

04 Once all of the tubes are filled, pour the remaining tomato sauce over the top of the pasta, then scatter over the grated mozzarella, if using.

Zhuzh it Up!
For some extra punch, add a couple of cloves of fresh crushed garlic to the spinach and ricotta mixture before filling the cannelloni tubes.

TO COOK: Simply transfer to an oven preheated to 180°C/350°F/gas mark 4 for 30–40 minutes, until the top is golden and bubbling and the pasta is tender.

TO FREEZE: Cover the Cannelloni with a lid, or wrap in a layer of clingfilm followed by a layer of foil, then label and freeze flat for up to 1 month.

TO COOK FROM FROZEN: This can be defrosted or cooked directly from frozen. If defrosted, cook as described left. If cooking from frozen, increase the cooking time to 1¼–1½ hours, covering with foil if the top starts to catch and ensuring it is piping hot before serving.

SPINACH & RICOTTA STUFFED CHICKEN

P

PREP: 10 MINS
COOK: 40 MINS
SERVES 4

8 cubes frozen, chopped
   spinach
1 x 250g tub ricotta
1 tsp ground nutmeg
4 skinless, boneless chicken
   breasts
8 slices Parma ham
salt and freshly ground
   black pepper, to taste

01 Put your frozen spinach in a heatproof bowl and cook in the microwave on high for 2½ minutes, then stir and cook for 2 minutes more. Drain the spinach through a colander lined with kitchen paper, pressing down to remove as much liquid as possible, then return the spinach to the bowl.

02 Add the ricotta cheese and nutmeg to the bowl with the spinach, then stir to combine. Season to taste and set aside.

03 Working with one piece of chicken at a time, place a chicken breast flat on a chopping board and press down with the palm of your hand. Working from the thickest end of the breast, insert a sharp knife two thirds of the way through the meat and carefully slice down the length to the thinnest end. Repeat until all your chicken breasts are butterflied.

04 Open your chicken breasts up along the cuts you have created and spoon a quarter of the filling mixture into each. Wrap each of the filled chicken breasts in two slices of Parma ham, securing as neatly as possible to keep the filling inside.

TO COOK: To cook straightaway, transfer to a foil-lined baking tray and cook in an oven preheated to 180°C/350°F/gas mark 4 for 30–40 minutes, until tender and juicy. Serve with your choice of vegetables alongside.

TO FREEZE: Lay the filled chicken breasts on a large sheet of foil, then fold over the edges and crimp together to form a sealed parcel. Transfer to a labelled freezer bag and freeze flat for up to 1 month.

TO COOK FROM FROZEN: Simply remove the chicken breasts from the freezer and leave to defrost fully, then cook as described left.

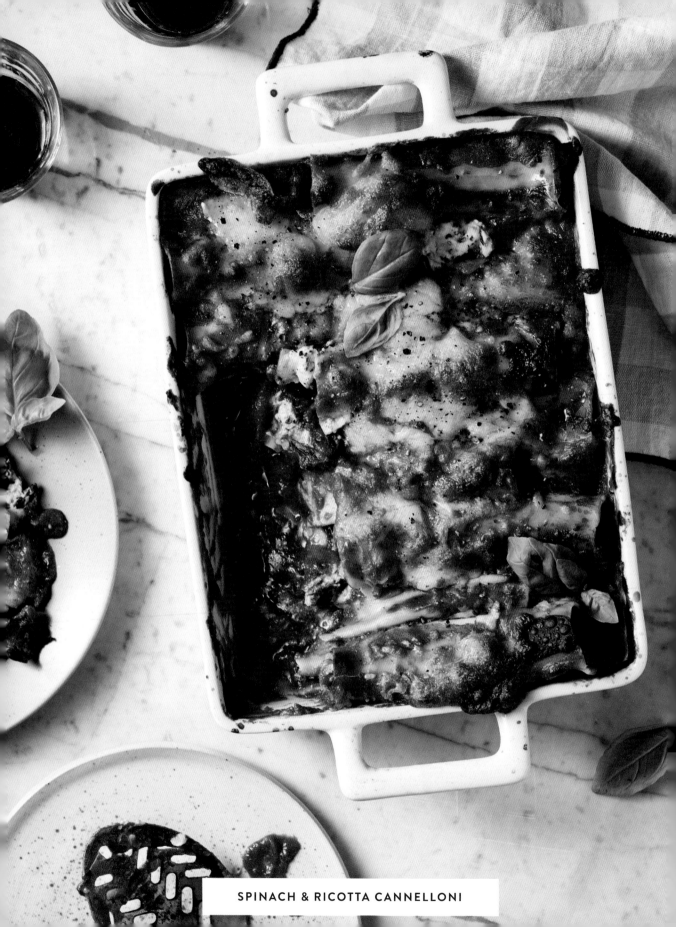

SPINACH & RICOTTA CANNELLONI

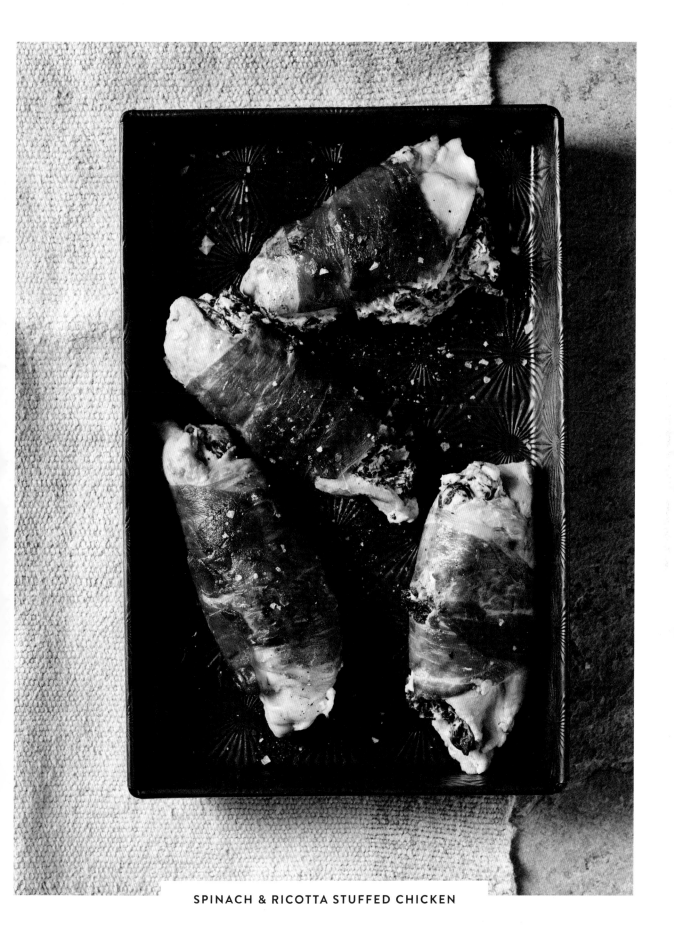

SPINACH & RICOTTA STUFFED CHICKEN

RUMBLEDETHUMPS

PREP: 15 MINUTES
COOK: 30 MINUTES
SERVES 4

2 cups (300g) frozen,
   chopped leeks
splash of olive oil
1 cup (115g) frozen,
   chopped onions
1 x 500g bag shredded
   cabbage or shredded
   mixed greens
1 knob butter
2 x 425g packs ready-
   made mashed potatoes
1½ cups (190g) grated
   cheddar cheese
20 cherry tomatoes,
   halved
salt and freshly ground
   pepper, to taste

If you've not heard of this, it's a classic Scottish dish that is delicious served as a side dish or even as the main event. The perfect meat-free comfort food for chilly winter nights! By using ready-chopped veg and pre-prepared mash, this dish can be assembled in moments.

01 Put the leeks in a heatproof bowl and cook in the microwave on high for 3 minutes, stirring halfway through cooking.

02 Heat the oil in a frying pan over a medium heat, then add the onion and cook, stirring, for 2–3 minutes, until softened.

If you are also making the Corned Beef Hash, cook the onions in the same pan now, then decant into a bowl and set aside while you continue with this recipe.

03 Add the leeks, cabbage or mixed greens to the pan along with a knob of butter and cook for 5–10 minutes, stirring occasionally, until the cabbage is tender and the leek and onions are starting to turn golden. Remove from the heat and tip the mixture into a large bowl.

While the cabbage is cooking, assemble your Corned Beef Hash.

04 Add the mashed potato and 1 cup (125g) of the cheese, then season to taste and stir until well combined. Now gently stir in the tomatoes, being careful not to break them up too much. Transfer the Rumbledethumps mixture to a large baking dish and flatten into an even layer.

TO COOK: Scatter the remaining cheese over the dish, then transfer to an oven preheated to 180°C/350°F/ gas mark 4 and cook for 20–25 minutes, until hot all the way through and golden and bubbling on top. Serve hot.

TO FREEZE: Cover with a lid or a layer of clingfilm followed by a layer of foil, then label and transfer to the freezer for up to 3 months.

TO COOK FROM FROZEN: This can be defrosted or cooked from frozen. If defrosted, cook as described, left. If frozen, cook for 1 hour, covered with foil for the first 45 minutes, then remove the foil and scatter over the cheese for the last 15 minutes.

CORNED BEEF HASH

Ⓜ

PREP: 10 MINUTES
COOK: 30 MINUTES
SERVES 4

splash of oil
2 cups (230g) frozen,
  chopped onions
1 x 340g tin corned beef,
  sliced
2 x 425g packs ready-
  made mashed potatoes
3 tbsp Worcestershire
  sauce
20 cherry tomatoes,
  halved

This simple classic is a childhood favourite of mine – a real Scottish winter warmer. Already a simple dish, I've made it even simpler by incorporating ready-made mash, which saves time and also freezes much better than homemade mashed potato. I love to serve this with pickled beetroot and oatcakes alongside, but my kids like to eat theirs with a big dollop of ketchup!

01 Heat the oil in a frying pan over a medium heat, then add the onion and cook, stirring continuously, for 5 minutes, until softened and starting to brown. Tip the cooked onions into a large bowl.

02 Add the corned beef, mashed potato and Worcestershire sauce to the bowl and use a potato masher to mash everything together until really well combined. Now gently stir in the tomatoes, being careful not to break them up too much. Transfer the hash mixture to a large baking dish and flatten into an even layer.

TO COOK: The dish can now be microwaved on high for 4 minutes, or transferred to an oven preheated to 180°C/350°F/gas mark 4 and cooked for 30 minutes, until hot all the way through.

TO FREEZE: Cover with a lid or a layer of clingfilm followed by a layer of foil, then label and transfer to the freezer for up to 3 months.

TO COOK FROM FROZEN: This can be defrosted or cooked from frozen. If defrosted, cook as described, left. If cooking from frozen, cook in an oven preheated to 180°C/350°F/gas mark 4 for 1 hour, covering with foil if the top starts to catch.

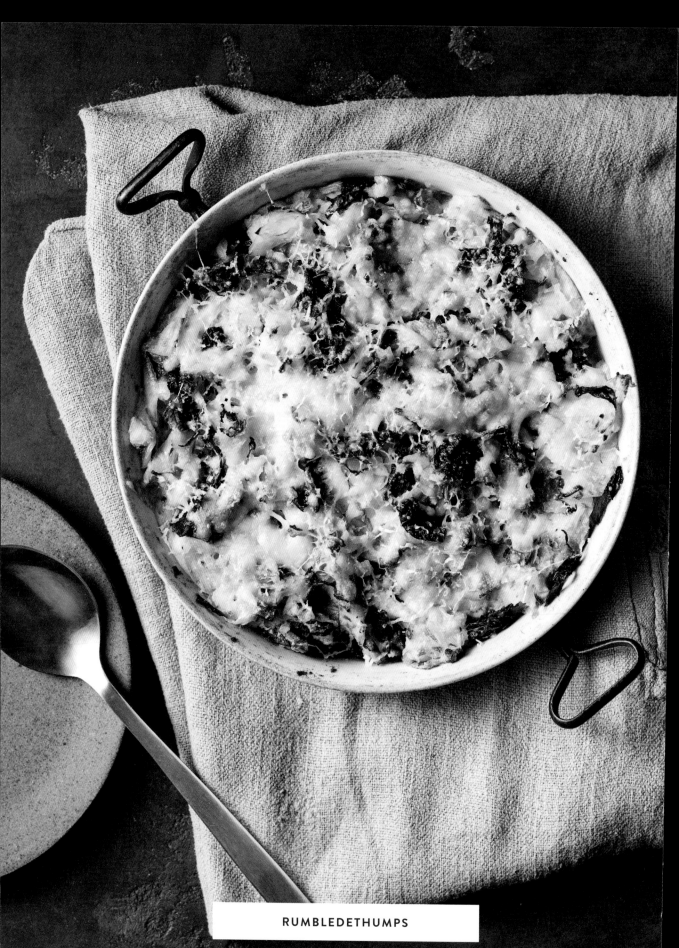

RUMBLEDETHUMPS

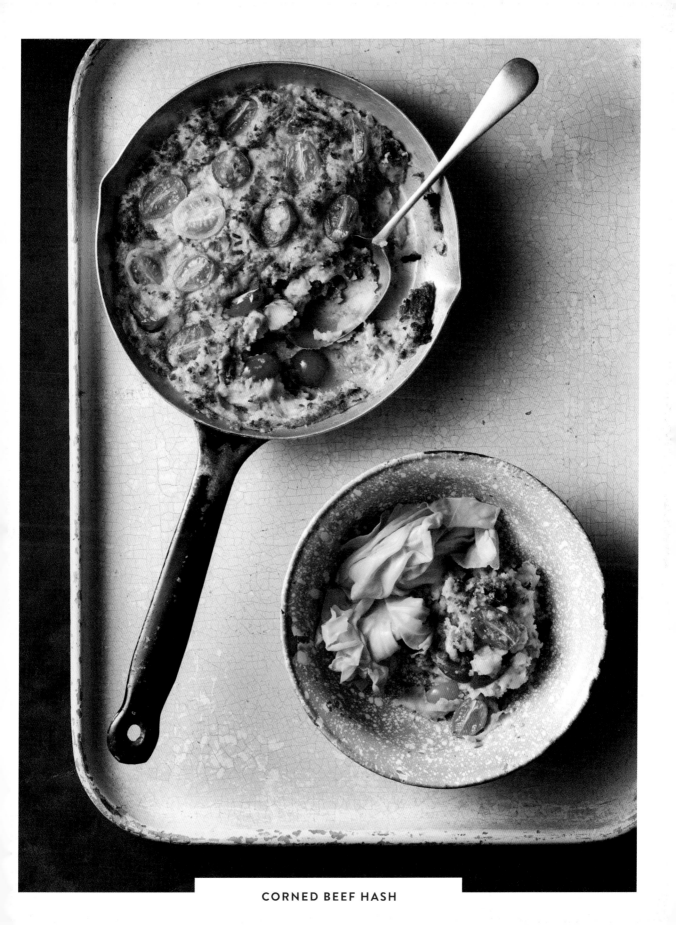

CORNED BEEF HASH

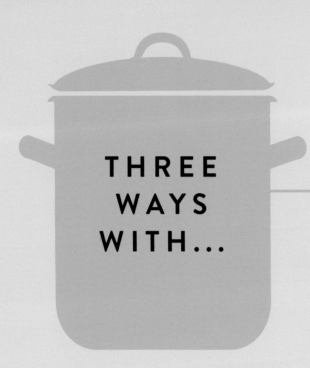

THREE WAYS WITH...

RUMBLE-DETHUMPS

Now that you've prepared your Rumbledethumps, what are you going to do with it? Below are three simple ideas for different ways of serving it that will keep meal times feeling fresh and different every time!

RUMBLEDETHUMPS WITH OATCAKES & BEETROOT

1 x quantity Rumbledethumps (p.164)
1 pack cooked beetroot, sliced, to serve
oatcakes, to serve

01 Prepare and cook the Rumbledethumps as per the recipe on page 164.

02 Divide the Rumbledethumps between four serving plates, then serve with a platter of oatcakes and sliced beetroot in the middle of the table, instructing your guests to add a spoonful of Rumbledethumps and a slice of beetroot to each oatcake.

Note
In Scotland, this is the traditional (and my favourite) way of serving Rumbledethumps.

RUMBLEDETHUMPS POTATO CAKES WITH PEAS

1 x quantity Rumbledethumps
  (p.164, made to the end of
  step 4 – see below)
1 egg, beaten
1½ cups (65g) panko
  breadcrumbs
3 cups (465g) frozen peas
salt and freshly ground pepper
splash of oil

01 Make the Rumbledethumps mixture to the
    end of step 4 as per the recipe on page 164,
    but do not transfer to a baking dish.
02 Set up a breading station by placing three
    bowls next to each other on the counter.
    Put the flour in the first, the eggs in the
    second and the breadcrumbs in the third.
    Season the flour with a generous grinding of
    salt and pepper and mix to combine. Lay a
    large sheet of greaseproof paper on the side
    next to the bowls.
03 Scoop out ½ cup of the Rumbledethumps
    mixture and form into a patty with your
    hands. Working as neatly as possible, dip it
    first in the flour to coat, then in the egg, then
    in the breadcrumbs. Once coated, set the
    potato cake on the sheet of greaseproof and
    continue until all of the mixture is used up.
04 Heat a splash of olive oil in a frying pan over
    a medium heat, then, working in batches, add
    the potato cakes and cook for 6–8 minutes
    on each side, until crisp, light golden and
    piping hot all the way through. While the
    cakes are cooking, cook the peas in boiling
    water as per packet instructions.
05 Divide the Rumbledethumps Potato Cakes
    between serving plates and serve hot with the
    peas alongside.

RUMBLEDETHUMPS WITH BAKED HAM & PARSLEY SAUCE

1 x quantity Rumbledethumps
  (p.164)
4 portions baked ham (buy
  slices from a butcher, or make
  your own – I have a good
  recipe on my website)
1 pack ready-made parsley
  sauce

01 Prepare and cook the Rumbledethumps as per
    the recipe on page 164.
02 While it is in the oven, carve the ham and
    heat the parsley sauce on the stove or in the
    microwave.
03 Divide the ham and Rumbledethumps
    between serving plates, then serve, passing a
    jug of the parsley sauce round for pouring.

OVEN-BAKED MUSHROOM RISOTTO

PREP: 10 MINUTES
COOK: 20 MINUTES
SERVES 4

25g butter
1 cup (115g) frozen, chopped onion
1½ cups (285g) risotto rice
½ cup (120ml) white wine
3 cups (720ml) vegetable stock
2 cups (140g) button mushrooms, roughly chopped
1 cup (80g) shop-bought grated Parmesan (use vegetarian Parmesan if you don't eat meat products)

This is a great basic risotto that is lovely as is, but can also be dressed up with chicken or fried cubes of pancetta, if you like.

If you are also making the Risotto Cakes, simply double the ingredients and use half of the finished Risotto to make the cakes.

01 Preheat the oven to 200°C/400°F/gas mark 6.

02 Melt the butter in a large, flameproof casserole or ovenproof pan over a medium heat, then add the onions and cook, stirring continuously, for 2–3 minutes, until soft.

03 Add the rice and cook for 2 minutes, stirring to coat in the butter, then add the wine and continue to stir until all the liquid has been absorbed. Pour in the stock and add the mushrooms, stir to combine, then transfer to the oven, covered with a lid, for 16–18 minutes.

While the Risotto is cooking, clear the sides and set up your breading station for the Risotto Cakes. This is also a good time to label any bags or dishes that you will be freezing the Risotto in.

04 Remove the Risotto from the oven and take off the lid – don't worry if the Risotto looks too liquid, it will start to thicken as you stir it. Add the Parmesan and stir through the Risotto.

TO SERVE: The Risotto can now be spooned into serving bowls and served hot.

TO FREEZE: Set the Risotto aside to cool to room temperature, then spoon into a labelled freezer bag and freeze flat for up to 3 months.

TO COOK FROM FROZEN: Defrost fully in the fridge. The Risotto can be transferred to a bowl and reheated in the microwave for around 3 minutes, until piping hot, or transferred to a pan and reheated on the stovetop until bubbling. If the consistency is too firm, simply add a splash of water to loosen.

PANKO RISOTTO CAKES

V

PREP: 15 MINUTES, PLUS COOLING
COOK: 20 MINUTES, PLUS MAKING THE RISOTTO
MAKES 16 CAKES, SERVING 8 PEOPLE

4 cups (960ml) Oven-baked Mushroom Risotto (recipe opposite)
½ cup (70g) flour
3 eggs, beaten
2½ cups (110g) panko breadcrumbs
4 tbsp olive oil
salt and freshly ground pepper
rocket salad, to serve

01 Make the Risotto as described on the opposite page, then pour onto a clean baking sheet and set aside to cool – for speed, this can be done in the fridge.

02 While the Risotto is cooling, set up your breading station by placing three bowls next to each other on the counter. Put the flour in the first, the eggs in the second and the breadcrumbs in the third. Season the flour with a generous grinding of salt and pepper and mix to combine. Lay a large sheet of greaseproof paper on the side next to the bowls.

03 Once the Risotto has cooled to room temperature, use an ice cream scoop to roll sixteen balls of the mixture. Set the scoops of mixture next to each other on the sheet of greaseproof paper.

04 Working with your hands, pick up a scoop of the Risotto mixture and flatten it gently to form a thick patty. Working as neatly as possible, dip it first in the flour to coat, then in the egg, and, finally, in the breadcrumbs. Once coated, set the Risotto Cake back on the sheet of greaseproof and continue the process until you have four coated Risotto Cakes.

05 Heat the olive oil in a frying pan over a medium heat, then add the Risotto Cakes and cook for 4 minutes on each side, until light golden and crisp. While the cakes are cooking, continue coating the remaining balls of Risotto mixture. Continue in this way until all of the Risotto Cakes are coated and cooked.

TO SERVE: The Risotto Cakes are now ready to serve. I like to serve two per portion with a lightly dressed rocket salad on the side.

TO FREEZE: Set aside to cool to room temperature, then transfer to a labelled freezer bag and freeze flat for up to 3 months.

TO COOK FROM FROZEN: These can be defrosted in the fridge or cooked from frozen. If defrosted, simply lay on a baking sheet and transfer to an oven preheated to 180°C/350°F/gas mark 4 for 15 minutes. If cooking from frozen, increase the cooking time to 30 minutes.

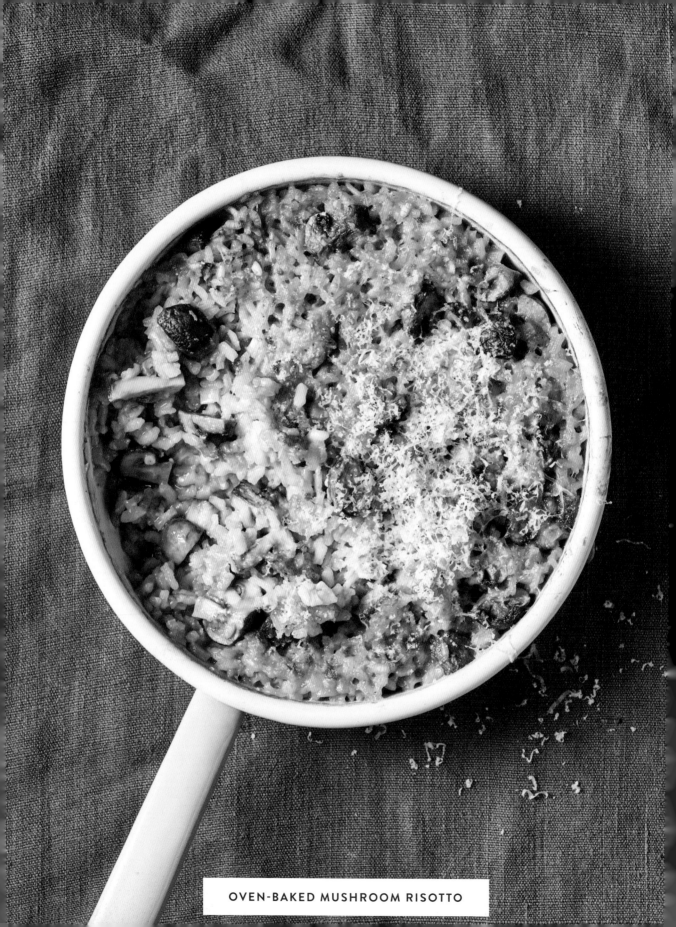

OVEN-BAKED MUSHROOM RISOTTO

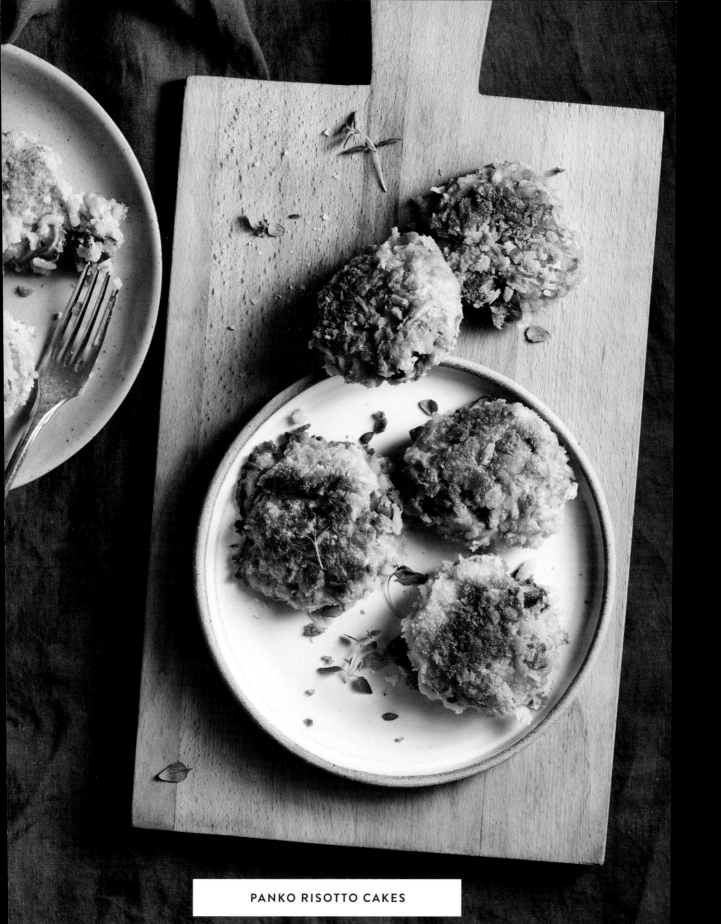

PANKO RISOTTO CAKES

OVEN-BAKED PEA RISOTTO

PREP: 10 MINUTES
COOK: 25 MINUTES
SERVES 4–6

5 cups (1.2 litres) vegetable stock
3 cups (465g) frozen peas
100g butter, cubed
2 tsp frozen, chopped garlic
10 spring onions, cut into 1cm (½ in) slices
2 cups (300g) Arborio risotto rice
1½ cups (150g) shop-bought grated Parmesan (use vegetarian Parmesan if you don't eat meat products)

This Risotto and the Pea & Mint Soup (opposite) are easy to make together as they use very similar ingredients and equipment, which also saves on the washing up! Simply whip up the soup while the Risotto is in the oven.

01 Preheat the oven to 180°C/350°F/gas mark 4. Put the vegetable stock and half of the peas in a large, ovenproof pan over a medium-high heat, bring to a boil and cook for 5 minutes.

02 Pour the stock and pea mixture into a blender and blend until smooth. Set aside.

03 Return the same pan to a low heat and add the butter, stirring occasionally until melted. Add the garlic and spring onions and stir to coat in the butter, then pour in the risotto rice and cook, stirring continuously, for 2 minutes until the grains are well coated in the butter.

04 Pour the pea and stock mixture back into the pan and stir to combine with the rice, then put a lid on the pan and transfer to the oven for 18 minutes, until the rice has swelled up and most of the liquid has been absorbed.

While the Risotto is cooking, make the Pea & Mint soup. To save on washing up, I use the same pan and blender jug for both dishes.

05 Remove the risotto from the oven and give it a quick stir, then add the remaining peas and stir through. Add the grated Parmesan to the pan and stir to combine, then cover and set aside for 2–3 minutes to thicken.

TO SERVE: Spoon the Risotto into serving bowls and serve warm. I like to serve this with a beautifully fresh lemon and rocket salad alongside.

TO FREEZE: Set the Risotto aside to cool to room temperature, then spoon into a labelled freezer bag and freeze flat for up to 3 months.

TO COOK FROM FROZEN: After defrosting fully, transfer to a bowl and reheat in the microwave for 3 minutes, until piping hot, or reheat on the stovetop until bubbling. If the consistency is too firm, simply add a splash of water to loosen.

PEA & MINT SOUP

PREP: 10 MINUTES
COOK: 10 MINUTES
SERVES 4

1 tbsp olive oil
1 cup (115g) frozen,
   chopped onion
1 tsp frozen, chopped garlic
1¾cups (420ml) chicken or
   vegetable stock
2 cups (310g) frozen peas
½ cup (25g) fresh mint
   leaves, chopped
½ cup (120 ml) double
   cream
freshly ground black
   pepper, to taste

01 Heat the oil in a large pan over a medium heat, then add the onion and garlic and cook, stirring occasionally, for 2–3 minutes, until soft.

02 Add the stock, peas, mint and a generous grinding of black pepper and stir to combine. Bring the mixture to a boil, then reduce to a simmer and leave to cook for 10 minutes.

This is a perfect time to wash up and clear down the sides, ready for packaging up your recipe for the freezer. (Don't wash the blender yet as you will need it for the next step.)

03 Pour the mixture into a blender along with the cream, then blend until smooth.

TO SERVE: Ladle the soup into serving bowls and serve warm. Perfect with a fresh, crusty roll alongside.

TO FREEZE: Set the soup aside until cooled to room temperature, then ladle into a large, labelled freezer bag, seal and freeze flat for up to 3 months.

TO COOK FROM FROZEN: Remove the bag from the freezer and leave to fully defrost in the fridge. Reheat the soup in a pan or microwave until piping hot.

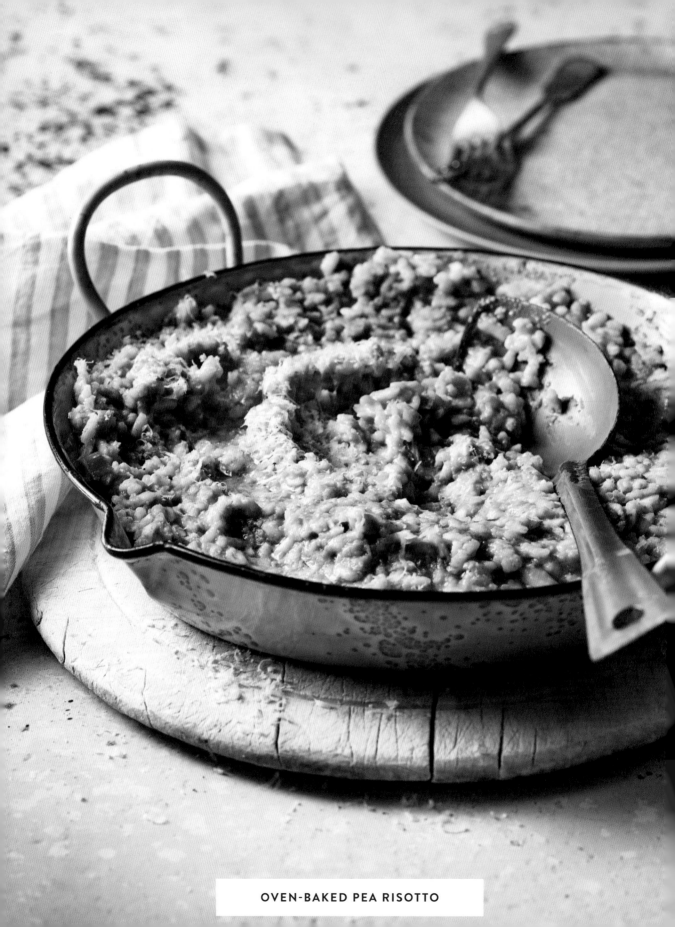

OVEN-BAKED PEA RISOTTO

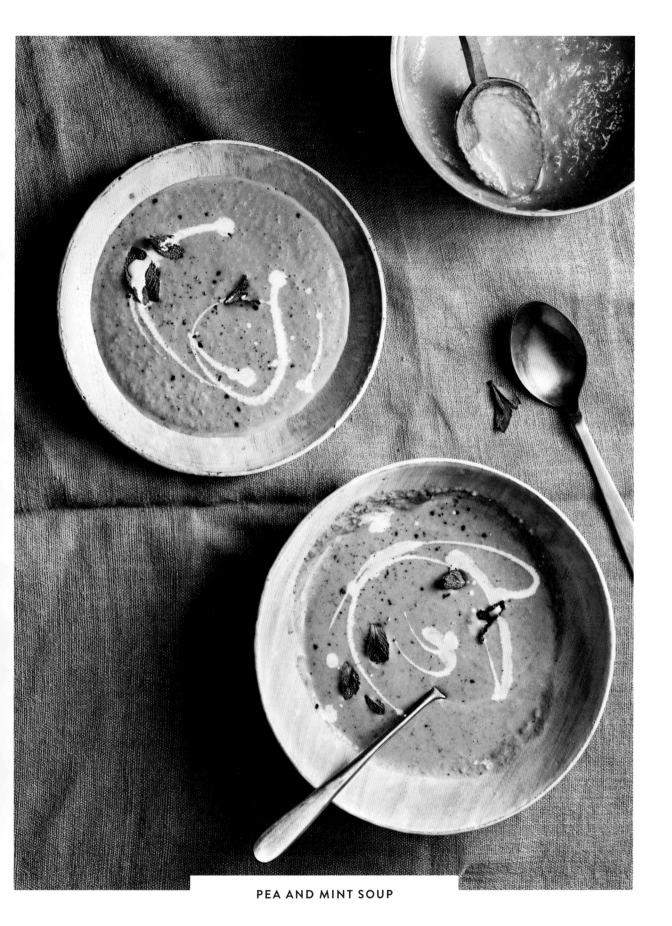

PEA AND MINT SOUP

10 MEAT-FREE MEALS IN 1 HOUR

Are you ready to cook ten meat-free family meals in just 60 minutes? This method includes some of my favourite veg dishes, such as Veggie Bolognese and Chilli Bean Burgers, which you can also find as individual recipes elsewhere in this chapter, though here they are scaled up to make a double portion and the methods are weaved together to make the best use of time. The recipes are a mixture of cooked and no-cook meals, so while one recipe is bubbling away, you can be prepping the next for the freezer.

The shopping list on the opposite page includes everything you need and I've scaled up the ingredients so you know what size pack to buy of each. Lay the ingredients out in piles according to the groupings overleaf, then follow the numbered guide and you can't go wrong!

Don't panic if this takes you more than an hour the first time you cook it – you will get quicker each time you make it. So, roll up your sleeves, get cooking and think about the time you'll be saving yourself in the future!

YOU WILL BE MAKING:

VEGGIE BOLOGNESE
VEGGIE CHILLI
VEGGIE FAJITAS
CHILLI BEAN BURGERS
STUFFED PEPPERS

SHOPPING LIST

Fresh

1 x 500g bag cubed root vegetables

14 fresh peppers (red, orange or yellow)

400g chopped mushrooms

4 fresh onions

4 fresh red onions

2 small bunches coriander

1 x 250g pack grated cheddar cheese

1 carton eggs

8 brioche burger buns (optional)

Frozen

1 x 75g bag frozen, chopped garlic

2 x 500g bags frozen, chopped onions

1 x 500g bag frozen, sliced peppers

1 x 700g pack frozen sweetcorn

Storecupboard

6 x 400g tins chopped tomatoes

4 x 500g cartons passata

5 x 400g tins kidney beans

2 x 400g tins black beans

2 x 400g tins three bean salad

1 x 180g tin sweetcorn

1 x 400g bag red lentils

1 bottle olive or vegetable oil

1 jar dried oregano

1 jar chilli powder

1 jar ground cumin

2 x 30g packs fajita seasoning

1 x 160g pack dried breadcrumbs

2 x 250g packs microwave rice

INGREDIENTS

GET ORGANIZED! Before you start make sure that your kitchen surfaces are cleared down, then lay all the ingredients out in individual piles according to the groupings on these two pages.

VEGGIE BOLOGNESE & VEGGIE CHILLI

For both dishes:
6 cups (300g) store-bought, cubed root vegetables (carrots, parsnips and swede work well)
splash of olive oil
4 cups (460g) frozen, chopped onions
8 tsp frozen, chopped garlic
4 x 400g tins chopped tomatoes
4 x 500g cartons passata
6 tsp dried oregano
400g red lentils, rinsed
For the Bolognese:
2 cups (140g) chopped mushrooms
For the Chilli:
4 tsp chilli powder
2 tsp cumin
2 cups (150g) frozen, sliced peppers
4 x 400g tins kidney beans, drained

VEGETABLE FAJITAS

2 x 400g tins black beans, drained and rinsed
4 cups (600g) frozen sweetcorn
2 x 30g packs fajita seasoning
4 fresh onions, peeled and thinly sliced
6 fresh peppers, deseeded and sliced
4 fresh red onions, peeled and thinly sliced

CHILLI BEAN BURGERS

2 x 400g tins three bean salad, drained and rinsed
1 x 400g tin kidney beans, drained and rinsed
2 cups (80g) breadcrumbs
1 cup (90g) tinned sweetcorn
2 eggs, beaten
3 tsp chilli powder
2 small bunches coriander, leaves chopped
8 brioche buns (optional)

STUFFED PEPPERS

8 fresh peppers, halved lengthways and deseeded
splash of olive oil
2 cups (230g) frozen, chopped onions
2 tsp frozen, chopped garlic
2 x 250g packs microwavable rice (choose your favourite flavour)
6 mushrooms, finely chopped
2 x 400g tins chopped tomatoes, drained through a sieve
2 cups (180g) grated cheddar cheese

METHOD

VEGGIE BOLOGNESE & VEGGIE CHILLI

01 Start by cooking the chopped root vegetables for the Bolognese and Chilli recipes in a microwave for 10 minutes, until just tender. Alternatively, cook in pan of boiling water over a medium heat.

02 While the vegetables are cooking, heat a splash of oil in a large pan over, then add the onions and garlic and cook, stirring, for 1 minute, until softened.

03 Add the chopped tomatoes, passata, oregano and lentils to the pan and stir to combine. Add the cooked root vegetables to the pan, too, then simmer for 20 minutes, stirring occasionally, until tender.

CHILLI BEAN BURGERS

04 While the Chilli and Bolognese are cooking, make the Burgers by putting both types of beans in a large bowl with the breadcrumbs, sweetcorn, eggs, chilli powder and coriander. Mix everything together with your hands until well combined, then divide the mixture into eight equal-sized balls.

05 Flatten the balls into patties, then transfer to a baking sheet lined with greaseproof paper – the burgers are fragile, so be careful when transferring them. Place the burgers in the freezer for up to 3 months, until ready to use. For ease, you can also freeze brioche buns to serve with your burgers; simply transfer the buns to a freezer bag and freeze flat.

VEGETABLE FAJITAS

06 Give the Bolognese and Chilli mixture a stir, then move on to preparing the Veggie Fajitas. You will be making two large freezer bags of fajita mixture, so set these on the side and remember to divide the ingredients between the two bags as you work. Put the ingredients into the bags in the order described, as you will need to cook them separately later.

07 Put half of the black beans and sweetcorn in each bag, followed by a quarter (half a pack) of the fajita seasoning. Next divide the peppers and onions between the bags and pour over the remaining fajita seasoning. Flatten the bags, removing as much air as possible, then transfer to the freezer until needed, up to 3 months.

08 To complete the Bolognese, place two large, clearly labelled freezer bags on the worktop and scoop four cups of the mixture into each. Now add 1 cup (70g) of the raw chopped mushrooms to each bag. Set the bags aside, unsealed, until the mixture has completely cooled, then seal flat and transfer to the freezer for up to 3 months, until needed.

09 The remaining mixture will form the basis of your Chilli. Simply stir the chilli powder, cumin, frozen sliced peppers and drained kidney beans through the mixture, then divide between two large, clearly labelled freezer bags. Set the bags aside, unsealed, until the mixture has completely cooled, then seal flat and transfer to the freezer for up to 3 months, until needed.

STUFFED PEPPERS

10 Finally, to prepare the Stuffed Peppers, put the halved peppers in a pan of boiling water over a medium-high heat and cook at a simmer for 4–6 minutes, until softened but still retaining their shape.

11 Meanwhile, heat a splash of olive oil in a frying pan over a medium heat, then add the frozen onions and garlic and cook, stirring, until softened – this should only take a minute.

12 Microwave your rice according to packet instructions – usually about 2 minutes – then add to the pan along with the chopped mushrooms, strained, chopped tomatoes and half of the grated cheddar cheese. Stir to combine, then remove the pan from the heat and set aside.

13 Drain the peppers and divide them between two baking dishes, packing them in to help them retain their shape. Spoon the filling mixture into the peppers, then sprinkle over the remaining cheese. Set aside to cool completely, then carefully wrap each of the peppers in clingfilm and transfer to a large freezer bag. Place in the freezer until needed, for up to 3 months.

Congratulations!
You now have 10 evening meals
ready for the freezer!

WHEN YOU COME TO COOK

Once cooked and frozen, all of these meals are best fully defrosted before cooking. All reheated meals should reach a temperature of 74°C/165°F. Always make sure any reheated food is piping hot before serving. Cooking times for each dish are listed below.

VEGGIE BOLOGNESE

Once defrosted, cook in a large pan over a medium heat, stirring occasionally, until piping hot and the mushrooms are cooked through. Alternatively, transfer to a heatproof bowl and cook in the microwave for 10 minutes, stirring halfway through cooking.

CHILLI BEAN BURGERS

Once defrosted, fry in a little oil for 3–4 minutes on each side. Alternatively, bake in an oven preheated to 200°C/400°F/gas mark 6 for 10–15 minutes, turning halfway through cooking.

VEGGIE CHILLI

Once defrosted, cook in a large pan over a medium heat, stirring occasionally, until piping hot. Alternatively, transfer to a heatproof bowl and cook in the microwave for 10 minutes, stirring halfway through cooking.

STUFFED PEPPERS

Remove the clingfilm from the peppers and layer in an ovenproof dish. Cook in an oven preheated to 180°C/350°F/gas mark 4 for 30–35 minutes, until piping hot and the cheese is golden and bubbling.

VEGETABLE FAJITAS

Once defrosted, fry the peppers and onions in a little oil until tender. While they are cooking, transfer the beans and sweetcorn to a heatproof bowl and cook in the microwave on high for 4 minutes. Stir the pepper and onion mixture into the bean and corn mixture and serve with tortilla wraps and your choice of toppings alongside.

SIDES &
SAUCES

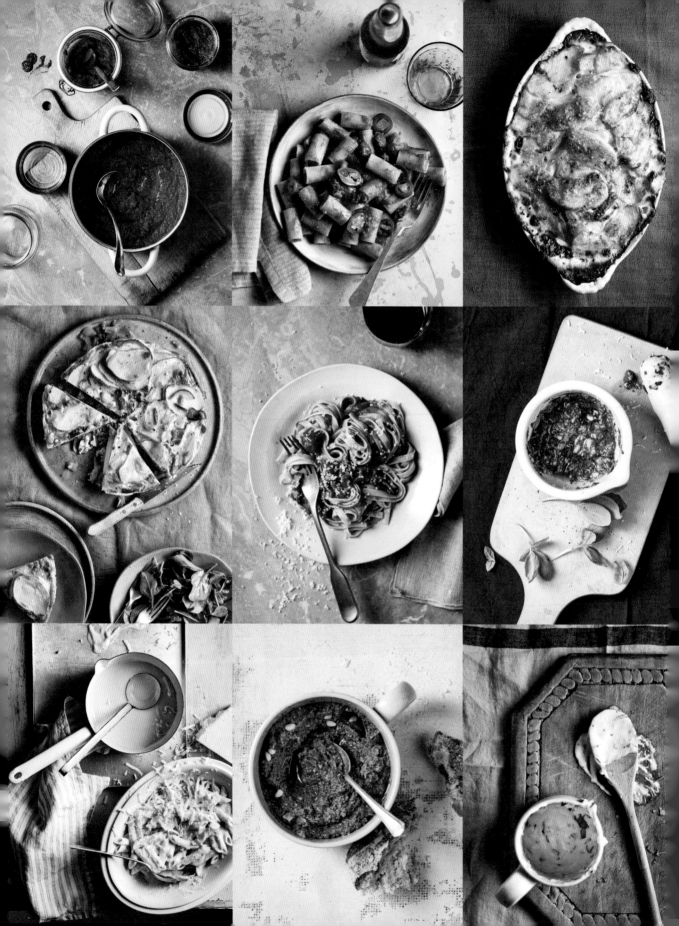

SIDES & SAUCES

Often overshadowed by the main event, with a little attention the humble side dish can be the star of the show! I like my veg to sparkle, so believe it's more than worth the time and effort to make your side dishes really shine. In this chapter you'll find recipes for all my favourite side dishes, from delicious Creamed Corn to indulgent Potato Dauphinoise.

Having these made ahead in the freezer, means that you can take out a main and a side at the same time and have a whole meal ready in no time. With a little planning, things that we all love but that normally take a long time to cook, such as roast or baked potatoes, can be whipped up in no time at all – bringing them into the remit of the midweek meal.

The sauces included in this chapter are all really versatile and freeze brilliantly. From recipes for Basic Tomato and Cheese Sauces to simple homemade pestos and more exotic enchilada and Alfredo sauces, you can have a host of ready-made sauces in your freezer that will transform a simple meal into something really special.

CREAMED CORN

PREP: 10 MINUTES
COOK: 15 MINUTES
SERVES 4

3 tbsp unsalted butter
2 tsp frozen, chopped garlic
½ tsp dried thyme
90g cream cheese
2 cups (300g) frozen
   sweetcorn
4 tbsp milk
salt and freshly ground
   pepper, to taste

This is a popular side dish in the US but relatively uncommon in the UK. If you're not familiar with it, then it's definitely worth trying as it's really delicious and a great way to zhuzh up frozen veg. I make a huge vat of it and freeze it in portions, but if you only have a small freezer you can easily freeze the sauce in small bags and add the sweetcorn to it after defrosting.

01 Preheat the oven to 190°C/375°F/gas mark 5.
02 Heat the butter in a pan over a medium heat, until melted, then add the garlic, thyme, cream cheese and a generous grinding of salt and pepper and stir to combine.
03 Add the sweetcorn to the pan, stir, then pour the mixture into a baking dish and transfer to the oven for 15 minutes, until thick, creamy and bubbling.

While the corn is in the oven, prepare the Chilli Green Beans.

TO SERVE: The Creamed Corn is now ready to serve. It goes brilliantly with fried chicken or makes the perfect side dish at a barbecue.

TO FREEZE: Set the dish aside to cool to room temperature, then cover with a lid, or wrap in a layer of clingfilm followed by a layer of foil, label and freeze for up to 3 months.

TO COOK FROM FROZEN: Remove the Creamed Corn from the freezer and leave to defrost fully in the fridge, then simply reheat for 3–5 minutes in the microwave, or heat in an oven preheated to 190°C/375°F/gas mark 5 for 10 minutes, until piping hot.

CHILLI GREEN BEANS

PREP: 5 MINUTES
COOK: 10 MINUTES

200g frozen green beans
splash of olive oil
1 tsp dried chilli flakes or
  frozen chopped chillies
salt, to taste

This is a great recipe for turning a simple green bean turn into a tasty side dish. If you're not a chilli lover, you can always substitute it for chopped garlic.

01 Cook the green beans in the microwave for approximately 4 minutes, until just tender but still retaining some bite. Drain through a colander to remove any excess water, then set aside.

02 Heat a splash of olive oil in a frying pan over a high heat, add the chilli flakes or crushed chillies and a generous pinch of salt and stir to coat in the oil, then tip in the green beans and cook, stirring, for around 5 minutes, until just starting to turn golden.

TO SERVE: The beans are now ready to serve. They make a great accompaniment to grilled fish or meats, or can be served alongside a warming stew or traybake.

189 SIDES & SAUCES

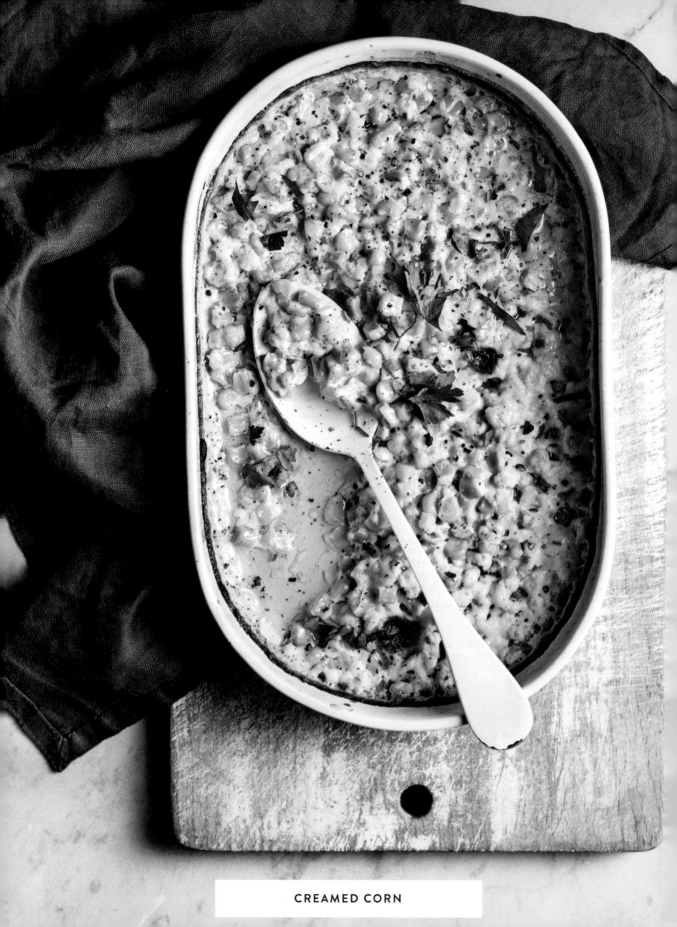

CREAMED CORN

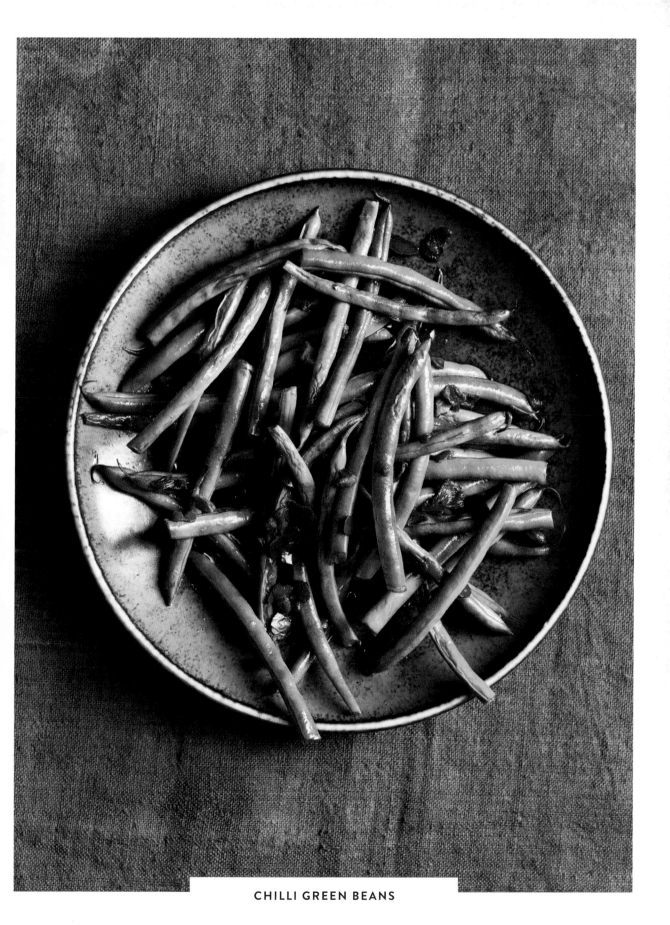

CHILLI GREEN BEANS

EASY ROAST POTATOES

PREP: 10 MINUTES
COOK: 55 MINUTES
SERVES 4

1kg potatoes (Maris Pipers work well), peeled and cut into quarters
½ cup (120ml) olive or sunflower oil
1 tbsp frozen, chopped rosemary (optional)
salt and freshly ground pepper

Zhuzh it Up!
For extra-special roasties, sprinkle these with chopped, fresh rosemary and a little sea salt before roasting.

Having roast potatoes frozen and ready to go means that you can just reach into the freezer and grab out however many you need. It also takes the stress and mess out of making a Sunday lunch, meaning that you can spend more time with your guests. This is one of the few instances where I will take the time to peel a potato. I've tried to roast potatoes unpeeled, but the result just isn't the same!

01 Line enough baking trays to lay all of the potatoes out flat with greaseproof paper and set on the side. Pour the oil into a large, shallow baking dish and add the rosemary, if using. Set aside.

02 Put the potatoes in a large pan of cold, salted water and place over a medium-high heat. Once boiling, reduce the heat to a simmer and leave to cook for 5 minutes, until just starting to soften at the edges.

While the potatoes are cooking, prepare the baking or sweet potatoes for the microwave.

03 Drain the potatoes through a colander, then leave for a few minutes to steam dry. Return the potatoes to the pan, cover with a lid and shake vigorously to fluff up the edges of the potatoes.

04 Working with a few potatoes at a time, lay the potatoes in the oil, turning to ensure they are fully coated, then transfer to the prepared baking sheets using a slotted spoon. Continue until all of the potatoes are coated in oil and laid out on trays.

TO COOK: Cook the potatoes in an oven preheated to 220°C/425°F/gas mark 7 for 45–50 minutes, turning halfway through cooking, until crisp and golden.

TO FREEZE: Set the potatoes aside until completely cool, then transfer to the freezer on their trays for 2 hours, until part frozen. After this time, transfer to large, labelled freezer bags, then return to the freezer for up to 3 months.

TO COOK FROM FROZEN: Remove the potatoes from the oven and transfer to a baking sheet, then cook in an oven preheated to 220°C/425°F/gas mark 7 for 45–50 minutes, turning halfway through cooking, until crisp and golden.

MADE-IN-ADVANCE BAKED POTATOES

PREP: 5 MINUTES
COOK: 30 MINUTES

4 tbsp sunflower or olive oil
1 tbsp salt
4 baking potatoes or large
  sweet potatoes, scored
  with a knife

Baked potatoes and baked sweet potatoes make a great, healthy midweek meal or side dish, but made fresh they take so long that there is rarely time to justify making them. I don't freeze these as they keep in the fridge for five days, so you can make them on a Monday and be eating them all week! They can simply be reheated in the oven for 10–15 minutes for perfect, deliciously fluffy interiors with golden, crispy skins.

01 Preheat the oven to 200°C/400°F/gas mark 6. Pour the oil into a baking dish and add the salt, then transfer to the oven to warm.

02 Put the potatoes in a heatproof bowl and cover with two layers of clingfilm, then cook in the microwave on high for about 15 minutes, checking after 10 minutes. You want them to be cooked through but not so soft that the skins are starting to wrinkle.

03 Once the potatoes are cooked remove the clingfilm, being careful to avoid the steam, then add to the tray in the oven, turning to coat in the oil. Leave to cook for 15 minutes, then turn and leave to cook until golden and crisp all over.

TO SERVE: The potatoes are now ready to serve, slathered in butter and filled with your choice of topping.

TO CHILL: These will keep in an airtight container in the fridge for up to 5 days.

TO COOK FROM FROZEN: The potatoes can be reheated in the microwave for 5–10 minutes or, if you want to crisp up the skin again, reheat in the oven at 200°C/400°F/gas mark 6 for 10–15 minutes.

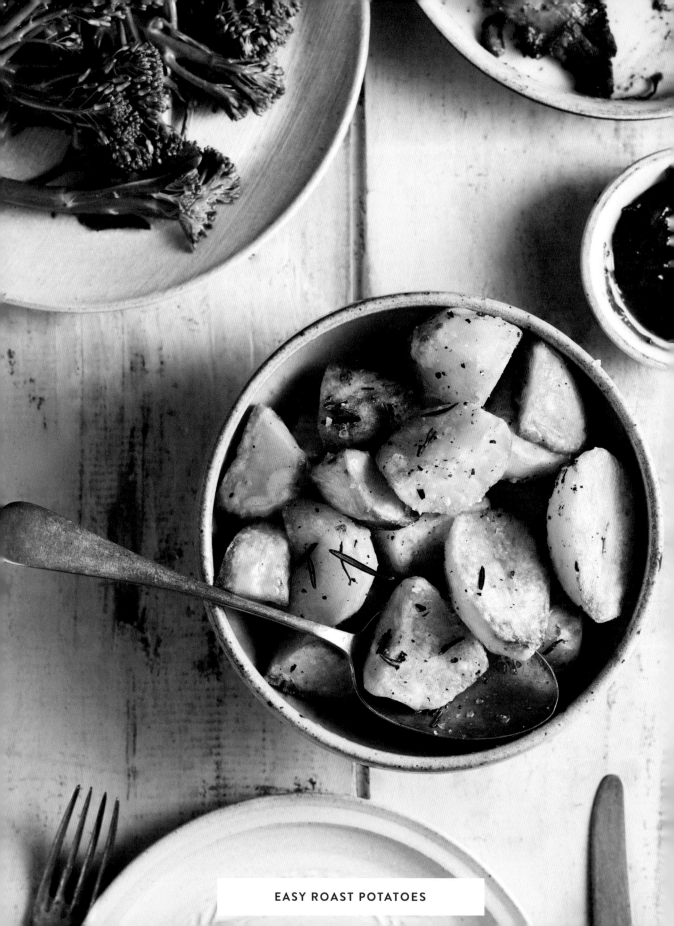

EASY ROAST POTATOES

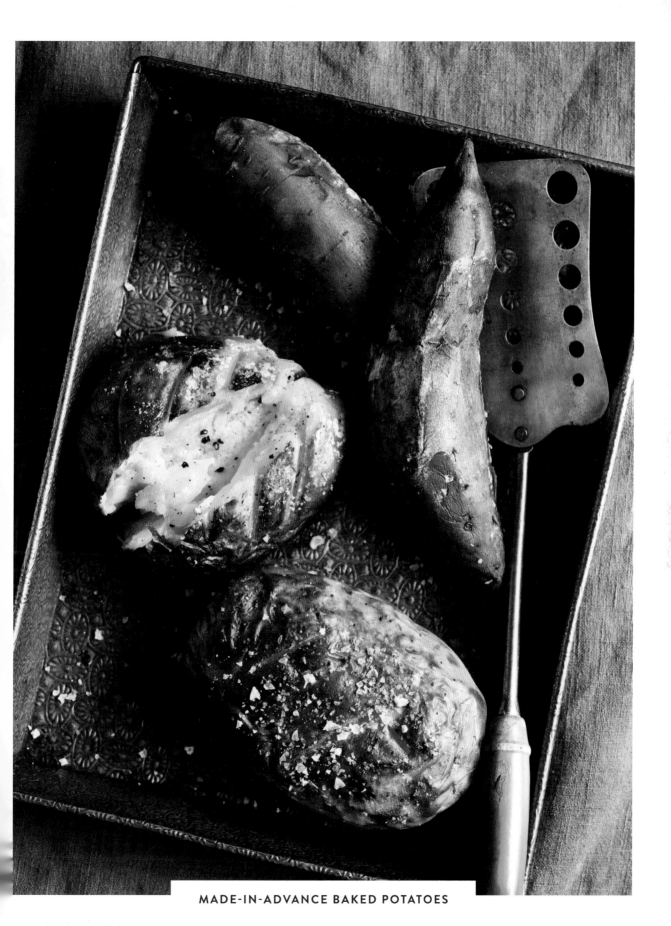

MADE-IN-ADVANCE BAKED POTATOES

POTATO DAUPHINOISE

PREP: 15 MINUTES
COOK: 30 MINUTES
SERVES 8

8 large potatoes (Maris
    Pipers work well)
2½ cups (600ml) double
    cream
1½ cups (360ml) whole
    milk
2 tsp frozen, chopped garlic
4 sprigs fresh rosemary
1 x 200g pack grated
    gruyere cheese
salt and freshly ground
    pepper

01 Preheat the oven to 180°C/350°F/gas mark 4 and grease a
    shallow baking dish with butter. Peel the potatoes and slice
    as thinly as possible, if possible using a mandolin or the slicing
    blade of a food processor.

*If you are also making the Spanish Omelette, slice the potatoes
for both dishes at the same time.*

02 Put the cream, milk, garlic and rosemary sprigs in a large pan
    with a generous grinding of salt and pepper and place over a low
    heat, stirring occasionally, until the mixture is warmed but not
    boiling. Add the potato slices to the pan, ensuring they are all
    submerged in the liquid, and leave to cook for 8–10 minutes,
    until just tender but still holding their shape.

Cook the potatoes for the Spanish Omelette in a different pan now.

03 Remove from the heat and pick out and discard the rosemary
    sprigs, then gently tip the mixture into the prepared baking
    dish, spreading out the potatoes so that they cover the surface
    in an even layer. Sprinkle the grated gruyere over, then bake in
    the oven for 20 minutes, until the potatoes are cooked and the
    sauce has thickened. If you are making these to freeze, remove
    from the oven before the top has browned as they will be baked
    again later. If you are making to eat now, leave until the top is
    beautifully golden and bubbling.

While the Dauphinoise is cooking, finish preparing your Spanish Omelette.

TO SERVE: The Dauphinoise is
ready to serve. It makes an ideal
accompaniment to roast meats
and vegetables, but a big bowl
on its own is also a deliciously
comforting treat!

TO FREEZE: Set aside until
cooled, then the Dauphinoise
can either be frozen whole or
cut into individual portions.
Either way, cover with a layer of
clingfilm followed by a layer of
foil, label and freeze flat for up
to 3 months.

TO COOK FROM FROZEN:
This can either be defrosted or
cooked from frozen. If defrosted,
bake at 180°C/350°F/gas mark
4 for 15–20 minutes. If frozen,
cook for 30 minutes, ensuring
that the Dauphinoise is piping
hot before serving.

SPANISH OMELETTE

V

PREP: 15 MINUTES
COOK: 30 MINUTES
SERVES 4

450g Maris Piper potatoes
splash of olive oil
1 cup (175g) frozen, sliced
   peppers
1 cup (115g) frozen,
   chopped red onion
6 large eggs, beaten
salt and freshly ground
   pepper

Zhuzh it Up!
Give this even more flavour by
adding in some chopped fresh
chilli, fresh herbs or thinly sliced
chorizo along with the peppers
and onions in step 3.

A delicious Spanish Omelette is a meal all in itself, but the slicing and boiling of potatoes can seem like a chore when you want to get something tasty on the table midweek. Made in advance and stored in the freezer, it can simply be defrosted and reheated for a comforting, no-fuss weekday meal.

01 Peel the potatoes and slice as thinly as possible, if possible using a mandolin or the slicing blade of a food processor. Bring a large pan of water to the boil, then add the potato slices, reduce to a gentle simmer and leave to cook for 8–10 minutes, until just tender but still holding their shape.

02 When the potatoes are almost finished cooking, heat a splash of olive oil in a frying pan, then add the peppers and onions and fry, stirring occasionally, until softened.

03 Drain the potatoes through a colander and set aside for a couple of minutes to steam dry, then add to the pan with the peppers and onions and stir to combine. Pour in the beaten eggs and season generously with salt and pepper, then leave to cook over a gentle heat for 10–15 minutes, until almost set.

04 While the omelette is cooking, preheat the grill to high. Then place the pan under the grill for 5 minutes to finish cooking the top.

TO SERVE: Set the Omelette aside for 5 minutes to firm up in the pan, then slide onto a large plate or chopping board. Cut into slices and serve warm with salad alongside. Any leftover Omelette will keep well in the fridge for up to 4 days.

TO FREEZE: Set the Omelette aside for 5 minutes to firm up in the pan, then slide onto a large sheet of foil. Allow to cool to room temperature, then wrap the Omelette in the foil, label and transfer to the freezer for up to 3 months.

TO COOK FROM FROZEN: Remove the Omelette from the freezer and leave to defrost completely in the fridge, then simply reheat in the oven or microwave until piping hot all the way through.

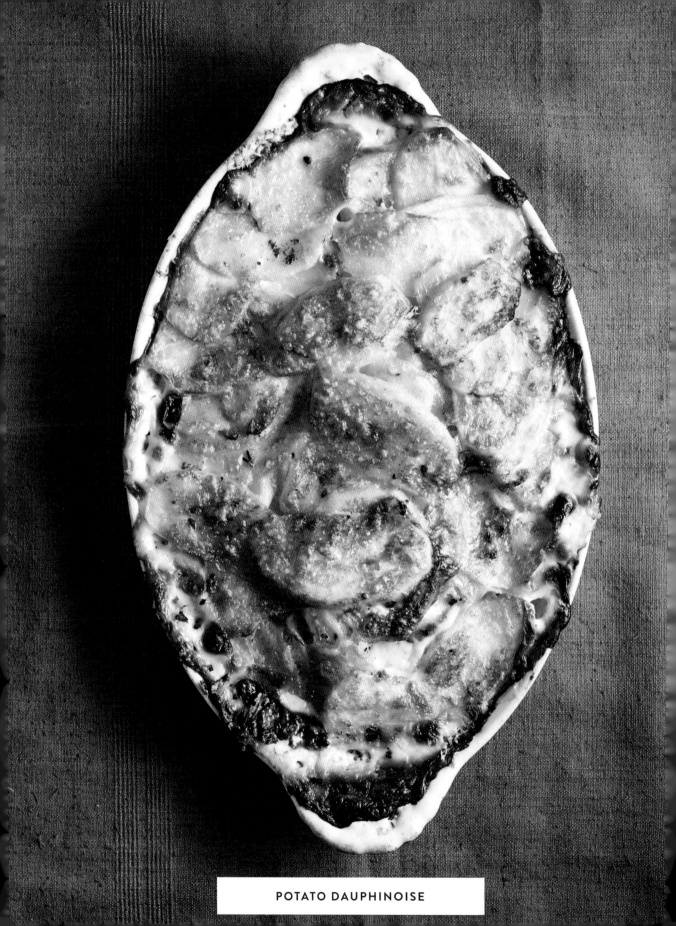

POTATO DAUPHINOISE

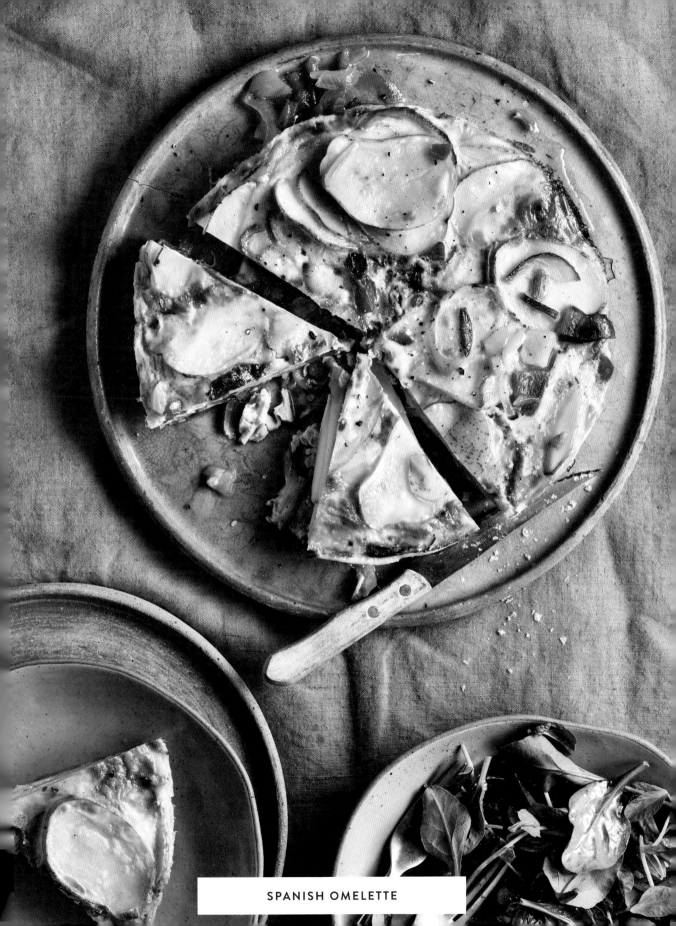

SPANISH OMELETTE

BASIC TOMATO SAUCE

PREP: 2 MINUTES
COOK: 15 MINUTES
SERVES 4

2 x 400g cans chopped
   tomatoes
1 x 500g carton passata
2 tbsp tomato purée
3 tsp dried oregano
1–2 tsp frozen, chopped
   garlic
salt and freshly ground
   pepper

If I am pushed for time, I am very happy to use a jarred tomato sauce at home. That said, this homemade version is very quick and kinder on the wallet than the store-bought variety. I like to make a big batch, then portion it out and keep in the freezer until needed.

01 To make the sauce, simply put all the ingredients in a pan over a medium heat and leave to simmer, stirring occasionally, for 15 minutes, until thickened.

If you are also making the Tomato-free Pasta Sauce, start that now while this sauce is cooking.

TO USE: The sauce is now ready to be used. It is great for dressing pasta, topping pizzas or using in any number of recipes, such as my Pepperoni Calzone (p.82).

TO FREEZE: Set aside to cool to room temperature, then transfer to a labelled freezer bag, seal and freeze flat for up to 3 months.

TO COOK FROM FROZEN: The sauce can be defrosted slowly in the fridge or more quickly in the microwave. Once defrosted, simply reheat till piping hot in a pan or in the microwave and use as described in the *To Use* section, left.

200 **THE BATCH LADY**

TOMATO-FREE PASTA SAUCE

PREP: 10 MINUTES
COOK: 15 MINUTES
SERVES 4

1 x 500g bag frozen, sliced
  carrots
splash of olive oil
2 cups (230g) frozen,
  chopped onions
4 tsp frozen, chopped
  garlic
4 store-bought, pre-
  cooked beetroot, roughly
  chopped
2 tbsp dried oregano
2 tbsp lemon juice
salt and freshly ground
  pepper

One of the recipes that people request most from me is a simple sauce that can be used to dress pasta or top pizza, that doesn't contain tomato. This is a great option if you have tomato-haters in your house, as the carrots add a sweetness to the sauce that is wonderfully balanced by the earthy flavour of the beetroot. This sauce is made in the blender, so make sure you have access to one before starting.

01 Bring a large pan of water to the boil over a medium heat, then add the carrots and cook for 8–10 minutes, until tender.

02 While the carrots are cooking, heat a splash of olive oil in a frying pan, then add the onions and garlic and cook, stirring, for 2–3 minutes, until softened.

03 Transfer the cooked onions and garlic to a blender along with the chopped beetroot, dried oregano, lemon juice and a generous grinding of salt and pepper. Once cooked, drain the carrots and add these to the blender along with 1 cup (240ml) of water. Blend the mixture until smooth, adding more water if the sauce is too thick (the desired thickness will depend on the sauce's intended use, for a pizza or calzone, the sauce should be thicker, for a Bolognese or lasagne, you will want a thinner sauce).

Note
If your blender is not large enough, simply process the ingredients in batches and combine at the end.

TO COOK: Pour the blended sauce into the same pan that the carrots were cooked in and place over a medium heat until bubbling. The sauce can now be used in place of classic tomato sauce in any of my recipes.

TO FREEZE: Set aside to cool to room temperature, then transfer to a labelled freezer bag, seal and freeze flat for up to 3 months.

TO COOK FROM FROZEN: The sauce can be defrosted slowly in the fridge or more quickly in the microwave. Once defrosted, simply reheat till piping hot in a pan or in the microwave and use as described in the *To Cook* section, left.

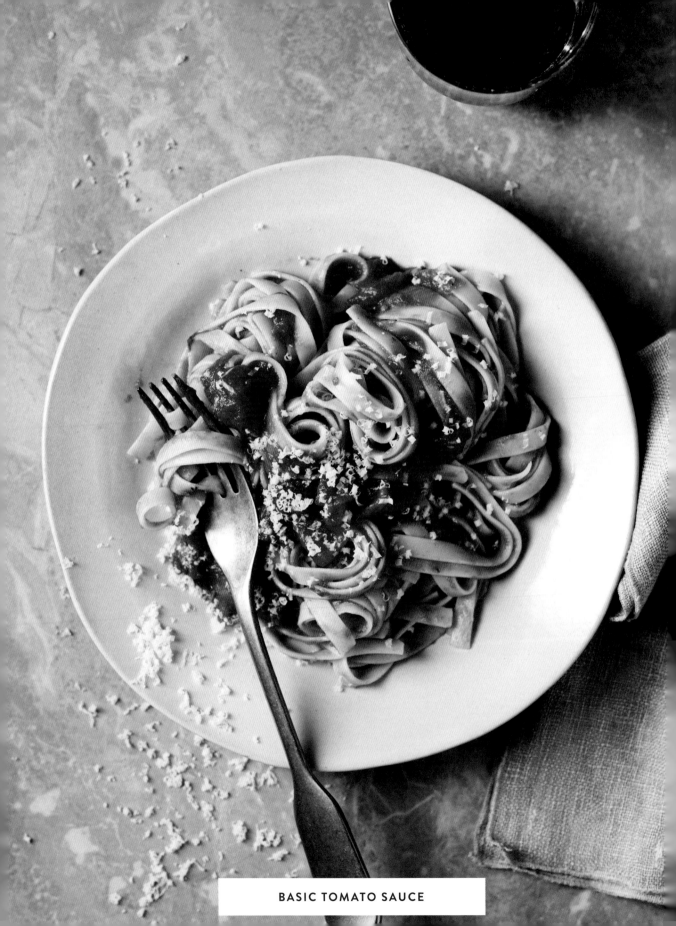

BASIC TOMATO SAUCE

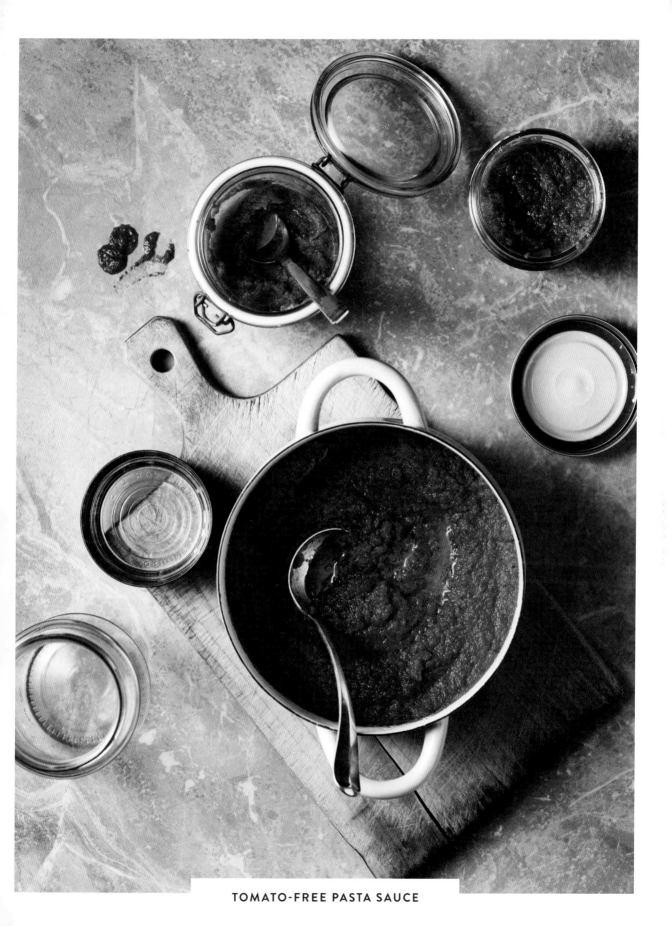

TOMATO-FREE PASTA SAUCE

THREE WAYS WITH...

BASIC TOMATO SAUCE

Now that you've prepared your Basic Tomato Sauce, what are you going to do with it? Below are some simple ideas for different ways of serving it that will keep mealtimes feeling fresh and different every time!

EASY TOMATO PASTA

2 cups (180g) dried pasta
   shapes of your choice
1 cup (240ml) Basic Tomato
   Sauce (p.200)
1 cup (90g) grated cheddar
   cheese

I will often make this recipe on a Sunday, then eat it throughout the week (it will last in the fridge for 5 days). It's great as an alternative to a sandwich for an easy, hot lunch and can be zhuzhed up with whatever other ingredients you need to be used up in the fridge.

01 Bring a large pan of water to the boil over a medium heat and add the pasta, then leave to cook according to packet instructions, until just tender. Drain and rinse the pasta through a colander, then return to the pan with the tomato sauce to heat through. Serve hot, garnished with grated cheese.

TOMATO PIZZA SAUCE

1 cup (240ml) Basic Tomato
  Sauce (p.200)
2 tbsp tomato purée
2 tsp dried basil
1 tsp frozen, chopped garlic

01 Simply put all the ingredients in a pan and
cook over a medium heat, stirring occasionally,
for 15–20 minutes, until thickened.

02 The sauce can now be used to top pizzas, or
left to cool then bagged and frozen for up to
3 months. I often freeze this with a ready-
rolled pizza dough alongside, so that I can
remove both from the freezer at the same
time for an easy supper.

OTHER USES FOR TOMATO SAUCE

Rather than give you a third recipe, I thought it
would be useful to list the recipes in this book
that you can use this sauce in. In these recipes,
simply omit any tomato sauce, passata, tomato
purée and Italian seasoning and use your ready-
made sauce instead.

- Lazy Lasagne (p.102)
- Mozzarella-stuffed Meatballs (p.103)
- Spinach & Ricotta Cannelloni (p.160)
- Pepperoni Calzone (p.82)
- Moussaka (p.205)
- Veggie Bolognese (p.86)
- Baked Sausage Ziti (p.78)
- Baked Spinach Ziti (p.79)

S

WHITE SAUCE

PREP: 15 MINUTES
MAKES ABOUT
2½ CUPS (600ML)

2½ cups (600ml) whole or
  semi-skimmed milk
½ teaspoon ground nutmeg
50g butter, cubed
4 tbsp plain flour
salt and freshly ground
  pepper, to taste

A classic white sauce or roux is one of those deceptively simple things that can feel quite intimidating to those who haven't tried it before. I have to admit, if I only need a small amount for a recipe then I will happily fall back on the store-bought, jarred variety, but when I am cooking in bulk, this is the recipe I use.

If you are making this and the Cheese Sauce recipe at the same time, you can start both in the same pan. Simply double the amount of butter, milk and flour and follow the steps below to make the basic sauce (omitting the nutmeg), then divide the mixture into two pans, adding the nutmeg to one to create the White Sauce and the mustard and the cheese to the other for the Cheese Sauce.

01 Put the milk, nutmeg and a generous grinding of salt and pepper in a jug and whisk to combine. Set aside.

02 Heat the butter in a large pan over a medium heat, until melted, then add the flour and cook, stirring, until the mixture has come together and thickened. Pour in a little of the milk mixture and cook, whisking continuously, until the liquid thickens. Keep adding more of the milk mixture to the pan, whisking and thickening between each addition, until all of the milk has been used up and you have a thick, glossy white sauce.

TO USE: The sauce is now ready to be used to make any number of dishes. I tend to make a big batch for when I am making several lasagnes and macaroni cheeses at once – this volume of sauce is enough to make three of either.

TO FREEZE: Set aside to cool completely, then ladle into a labelled freezer bag and freeze flat for up to 3 months.

TO USE FROM FROZEN: Remove the bag from the freezer and allow to defrost fully in the fridge, then reheat in a pan until bubbling and use as described in the *To Use* section, left.

CHEESE SAUCE

PREP: 15 MINUTES
MAKES ABOUT
2½ CUPS (600ML)

50g butter, cubed
4 tbsp plain flour
2½ cups (600ml) whole or
  semi-skimmed milk
2 cups (180g) grated
  cheddar cheese
1 tsp Dijon mustard
  (optional)

01 Heat the butter in a large pan over a medium heat, until melted, then add the flour and cook, stirring, until the mixture has come together and thickened. Pour in a little of the milk and cook, whisking continuously, until the liquid has thickened. Keep adding more of the milk to the pan, whisking and thickening between each addition, until all of the milk has been used up and you have a thick, glossy white sauce.

02 Remove the pan from the heat and add the cheese and Dijon mustard, if using, then whisk until the cheese has melted into the sauce.

TO USE: The sauce is now ready to be used to make any number of dishes. It is great served over cooked chicken or baked in a cauliflower cheese. It can also be used to make moussaka, lasagne or macaroni cheese.

TO FREEZE: Set aside to cool completely, then ladle into a labelled freezer bag and freeze flat for up to 3 months.

TO USE FROM FROZEN: Remove the bag from the freezer and allow to defrost fully in the fridge, then reheat in a pan until bubbling and use as described in the *To Use* section, left.

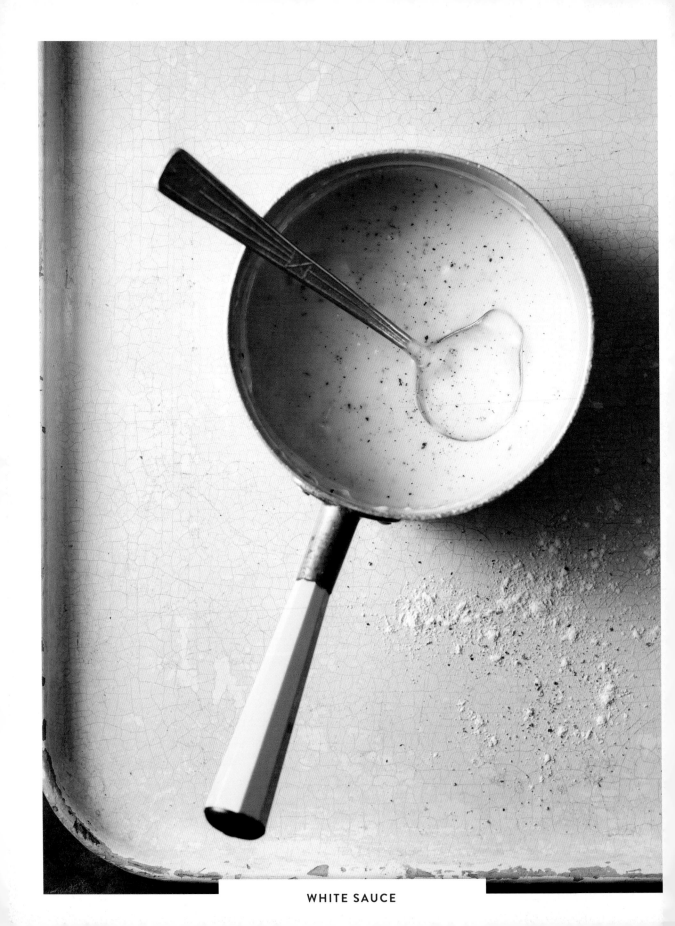

WHITE SAUCE

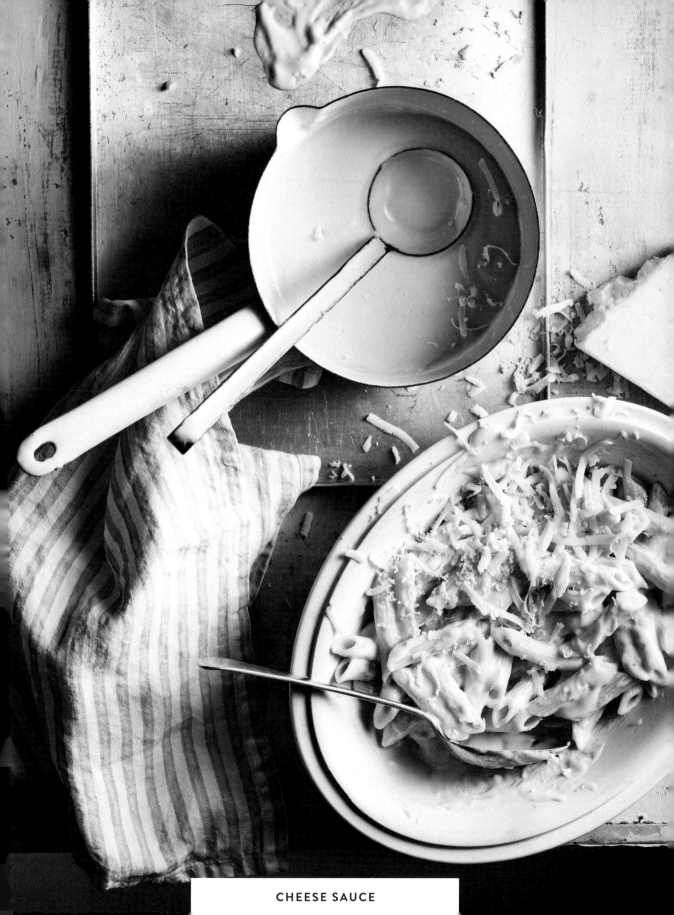

CHEESE SAUCE

ALFREDO SAUCE

PREP: 15 MINUTES
MAKES 1 CUP (240ML)

¼ cup (60g) butter
1 cup (240ml) double
  cream
2 tsp frozen, chopped garlic
1⅓ cups (150g) grated
  gruyere cheese
¼ cup chopped fresh
  parsley (optional)

A little of this rich and creamy sauce goes a long way. It's really versatile, freezes well and is also the basis of my Alfredo Chicken Pasta Bake (see opposite) – I like to make a big batch of sauce so that I can assemble the bake and still have plenty left over to use as a coating for pasta, to top pizzas or to dress up a simple cooked chicken breast.

If you are making the Alfredo Chicken Pasta Bake, put the pasta on now while you make the sauce.

01 Place the butter in a saucepan over a medium-to-low heat. Once melted, add the cream and stir continuously until the sauce starts to thicken, about 5 minutes.

02 Add the garlic and cheese to the pan and continue to stir until the cheese has melted into the sauce. Stir through the parsley, if using, then remove the pan from the heat.

Zhuzh it Up!
For a special supper, add a couple of crushed cloves of garlic to the sauce and serve stirred through linguine and topped with cooked prawns.

TO COOK: The sauce can now be used to dress pasta, top pizzas or spooned over cooked meats or vegetables before serving.

TO FREEZE: If making the sauce to freeze for later, leave it to cool to room temperature, then transfer to a sealable freezer bag, label and seal flat. Freeze for up to 3 months.

TO COOK FROM FROZEN: Allow to defrost fully in the fridge, then transfer to saucepan and cook over a low-to-medium heat, stirring, until piping hot. The sauce is now ready to use.

ALFREDO CHICKEN PASTA BAKE

PREP: 20 MINUTES
COOK: 25 MINUTES
SERVES 4

3 cups (250g) dried penne
splash of olive oil
3 chicken breasts, cut into
    5mm (¼ in) slices
1 cup (115g) frozen,
    chopped onions
1 head broccoli, cut into
    small florets
1 x quantity Alfredo Sauce
    (see opposite)
1 x 180g tub cream cheese
1 cup (90g) grated cheese
2 cups (220g)
    breadcrumbs

01 Put the pasta in a large saucepan and pour over boiling water to cover, place over a medium-high heat and bring to the boil. Reduce the heat to a simmer and leave to cook according to packet instructions, until al dente.

> If you have not yet made the Alfredo Sauce, make it now while the pasta finishes cooking.

02 Heat a splash of olive oil in a frying pan over a medium heat, then add the chicken and onions and cook, stirring, for 3–4 minutes, until the chicken is cooked through. Set aside.

03 Place the broccoli florets in a heatproof bowl with 3 tablespoons of water and cover with clingfilm or a large plate. Microwave the broccoli on high for 3–4 minutes, until just tender but still retaining some bite.

04 Once cooked, drain and rinse the pasta, then return to the pan. Add the Alfredo Sauce and cream cheese and stir until the pasta is nicely coated and the cheese has melted into the sauce. Now add the cooked chicken and onion mixture along with the broccoli and stir again until well combined.

05 Transfer the mixture to a large ovenproof or disposable foil dish, then scatter over the grated cheese and breadcrumbs.

TO COOK: Transfer to an oven preheated to 200°C/400°F/ gas mark 6 and cook for 20–25 minutes, until golden brown and bubbling. Serve immediately.

TO FREEZE: If making to freeze for later, set aside to cool to room temperature, then cover with a layer of clingfilm followed by a layer of foil, label and freeze. This will keep in the freezer for up to 3 months.

TO COOK FROM FROZEN: Remove from the freezer and leave to fully defrost in the fridge. Once defrosted, simply follow the cooking instructions in the *To Cook* section, left.

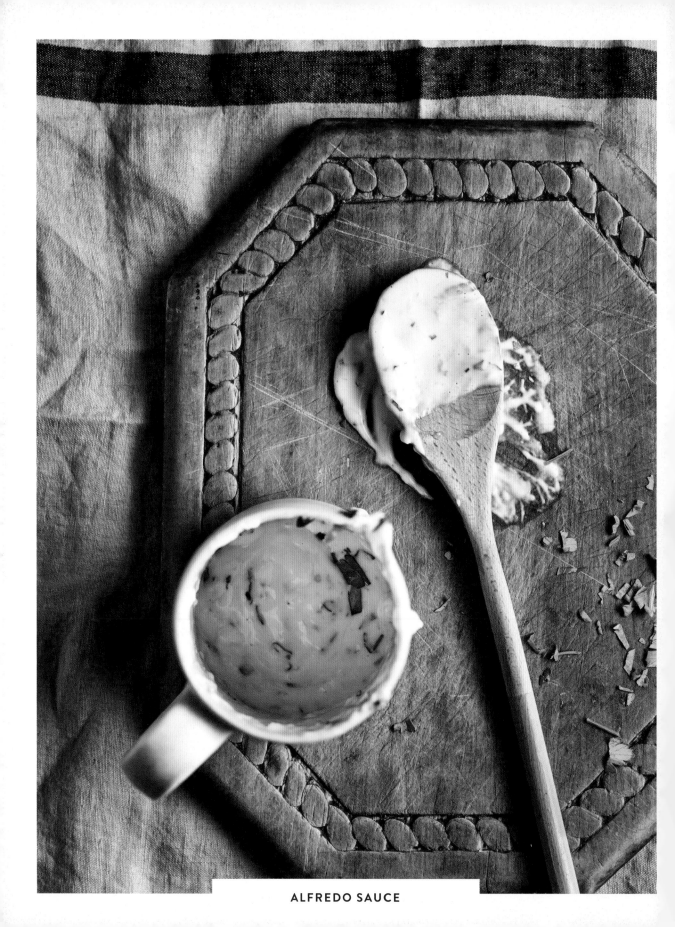

ALFREDO SAUCE

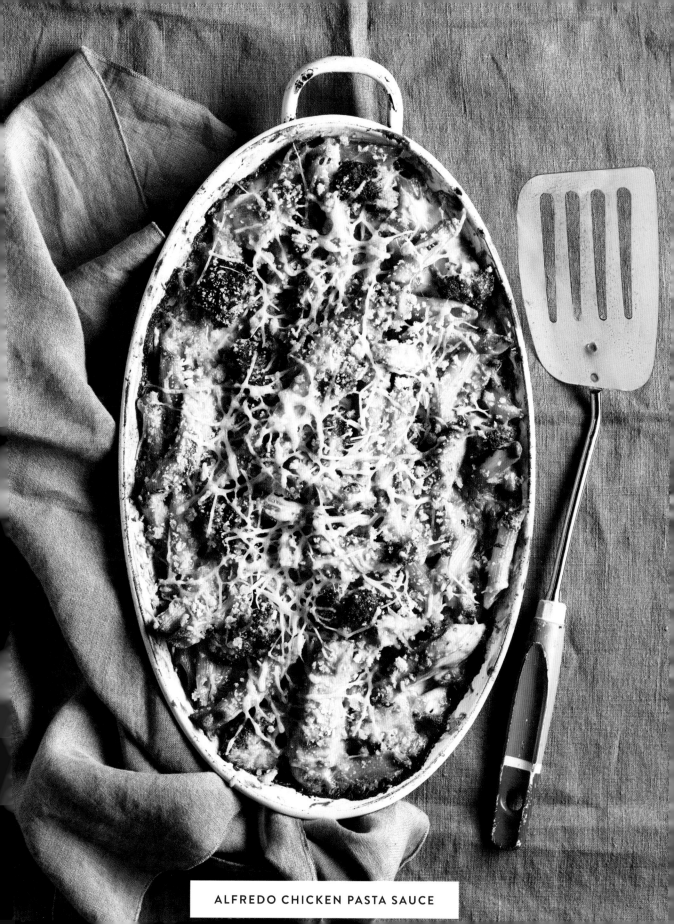

ALFREDO CHICKEN PASTA SAUCE

ENCHILADA PASTA SAUCE

PREP: 15 MINUTES
**MAKES ENOUGH
SAUCE FOR 2 MEALS,
EACH SERVING 4
PEOPLE**

2 tbsp vegetable oil
½ cup (60g) plain flour
2 x 580g cartons passata
2 x 30g packs fajita
    seasoning
splash of olive oil
1 cup (115g) frozen,
    chopped onions
1 cup (175g) frozen,
    chopped peppers
2 tbsp sliced jalapenos
1 cup (140g) frozen, diced
    chorizo (optional)

I love to have ready-made sauces on hand to pour over cooked pasta for an instant dinner. Pasta sauces are so easy to make that I always double the amount and freeze some for later.

01 Heat the oil in a small pan over a medium heat, then add the flour and cook, whisking continuously, to form a smooth, thick paste. Add the passata and fajita seasoning and continue whisking for 5–10 minutes until the mixture has thickened. Remove from the heat.

02 While you are thickening the sauce, heat a splash of oil in a frying pan over a medium heat, then add the onions, peppers, jalapenos and chorizo, if using, and cook, stirring occasionally, for around 5 minutes.

03 When the sauce has thickened, pour the mixture from the frying pan into the sauce and stir to combine.

Note
If you are vegetarian or cutting down on meat, simply omit the chorizo for a vegetarian Enchilada Sauce.

TO USE: The sauce is now ready to be used to dress pasta (I like it with rigatoni) or to make Baked Enchiladas (opposite).

TO FREEZE: Set the sauce aside to cool to room temperature, then divide into two labelled freezer bags and freeze flat for up to 3 months.

TO COOK FROM FROZEN: Remove a bag of sauce from the freezer and allow to defrost fully in the fridge, then simply reheat the sauce in a pan or the microwave until piping hot and use as described in the *To Use* section, left.

BAKED ENCHILADAS

(V)

PREP: 15 MINUTES
COOK: 25 MINUTES
SERVES 4

splash of olive oil
1 cup (115g) frozen,
   chopped onions
1 tsp ground cumin
1 cup (140g) frozen
   sweetcorn
½ cup (150g) frozen,
   chopped peppers
1 x 400g can black beans,
   drained
1 cup (250g) tomato salsa
1 cup (115g) grated cheddar
   or mozzarella cheese
6 corn tortilla wraps
½ quantity Enchilada Pasta
   Sauce (p.214), made
   omitting the chorizo or
   1 large jar shop-bought
   enchilada sauce

If you don't include the chorizo in the Enchilada Sauce recipe, this makes a great meat-free, midweek meal. Because there are a couple of elements to prepare and a bit of assembly required, it may seem complicated at first, but this is actually a really simple, flavour-packed dish!

01 Heat a splash of oil in a pan over a medium heat, then add the onion and cumin and cook, stirring, for 2–3 minutes, until softened.

02 Add the sweetcorn, peppers, black beans and salsa to the pan and stir to combine. Once the mixture starts to bubble, reduce the heat to a simmer and leave to cook for 3–4 minutes.

If you have not yet made your Enchilada Pasta Sauce, start it now.

03 Add two-thirds of the grated cheese to the pan and stir to combine, then remove from the heat and set aside.

04 To assemble the enchiladas, heat the tortilla wraps in the microwave for 15 seconds, then spoon 4 tablespoons of the filling mixture and 4 tablespoons of the sauce into each one. Roll the tortillas around the filling and arrange, seam-side down, in a large baking dish. Repeat until all of the tortillas are used up, then pour any remaining sauce over the top of the Enchiladas and scatter over the remaining cheese.

TO COOK: Transfer the enchiladas to an oven preheated to 180°C/350°F/gas mark 4 and bake for 20 minutes, until the sauce is bubbling and the top is golden.

TO FREEZE: Leave the enchiladas to cool to room temperature, then cover with a lid or wrap in a layer of clingfilm followed by a layer of foil, label and freeze flat for up to 3 months.

TO COOK FROM FROZEN: These can be defrosted or cooked from frozen. If defrosted, follow the cooking instructions in the *To Cook* section, left. If frozen, cook for 40 minutes, covering with foil if the top starts to catch.

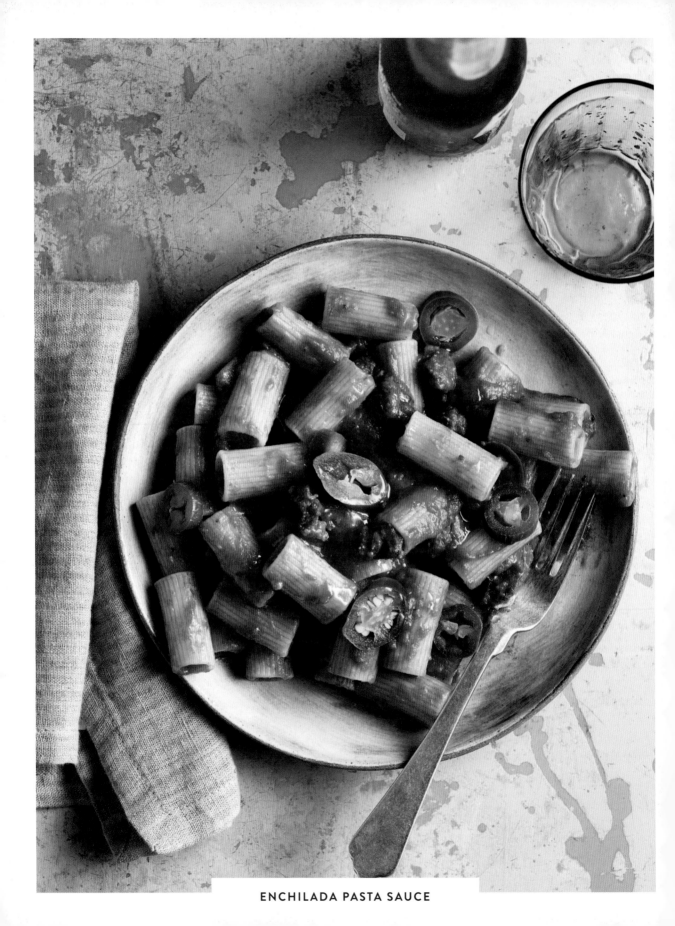

ENCHILADA PASTA SAUCE

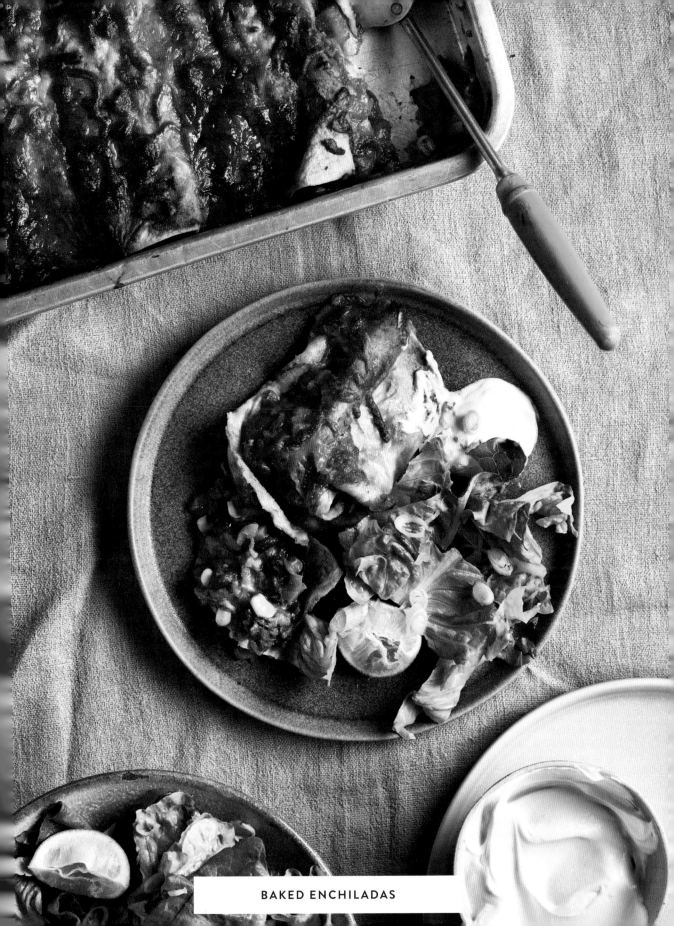

BAKED ENCHILADAS

THREE WAYS WITH...

ENCHILADA PASTA SAUCE

Now that you've prepared your Enchilada Pasta Sauce, what are you going to do with it? Below are three simple ideas for different ways of serving it that will keep mealtimes feeling fresh and different every time.

VEGETABLE ENCHILADA PASTA

2 cups (180g) dried penne pasta
splash of olive oil
2 cups (140g) sliced
  mushrooms
2 cups (480ml) Enchilada Pasta
  Sauce, made omitting the
  chorizo (p.214)

01 Bring a large pan of water to the boil, then add the pasta and cook for 10–12 minutes, until tender.

02 Heat a splash of olive oil in a frying pan over a medium heat, then add the mushrooms and cook, stirring, for 2–3 minutes, until tender. Add the pasta sauce and cook, stirring until bubbling.

03 Once the pasta is cooked, drain through a colander, return to the pan and pour the sauce and mushroom mixture over the top. Stir to combine, then divide the mixture into serving dishes and serve hot.

CLASSIC CHICKEN ENCHILADAS

splash of olive oil

3 skinless, boneless chicken
  breasts, sliced

2 peppers, sliced

4 corn tortilla wraps

2 cups (480ml) Enchilada
  Pasta Sauce (p.214)

1 cup (90g) grated cheddar
  cheese

01 Preheat the oven to 180°C/350°F/gas mark 4.

02 Heat a splash of olive oil in a frying pan over
    a medium heat, then add the chicken and
    peppers and cook, stirring occasionally,
    for 10–12 minutes, until the chicken is
    cooked through.

03 Heat the tortilla wraps in the microwave
    for 15 seconds, then spoon 2 tablespoons
    of the chicken and pepper mixture and 2
    tablespoons of the sauce into each one.
    Scatter a tablespoon of cheese over each,
    then roll the tortillas around the filling and
    arrange, seam-side down, in a large baking
    dish. Repeat until all of the tortillas are used
    up, then pour any remaining sauce over the
    top of the enchiladas and scatter over the
    remaining cheese.

04 Transfer to the oven and bake for 20–25
    minutes until golden and bubbling, then
    divide between 4 serving plates and serve hot.

ENCHILADA SAUCE & CRUDITÉS

2 cups (480ml) Enchilada
  Pasta Sauce (p.214)

sliced fresh peppers

carrot batons

tortilla chips

bread sticks

cheese batons

01 Put the sauce in a heatproof bowl and cook in
    the microwave for 2 minutes, until hot.

02 Serve the sauce with the vegetables, crisps
    and cheese served alongside for dipping. This
    is great as an informal appetizer for a party or
    a quick midweek dinner for the kids.

GREEN PESTO

PREP: 5 MINUTES
**MAKES ABOUT 1 CUP
(240ML)**

5 tbsp pine nuts
⅔ cup (160ml) olive oil
2 tsp frozen, chopped garlic
5 tbsp store-bought,
   grated Parmesan cheese
2 cups (about 60g) basil
   leaves
½ tsp salt

Making pesto is so simple to do but somehow makes me feel like a domestic goddess! Both this and the Red Pesto recipe (opposite) use similar ingredients, so why not knock up both batches at once?

01 Simply transfer all of the ingredients to a blender and blend to your desired consistency – depending on if you prefer a coarser or smoother pesto. If the mixture is too dry, simply add a little more oil.

TO USE: The pesto is now ready to use. It is delicious used to dress pasta or spooned over grilled fish or meats.

TO FREEZE: I like to freeze pesto in ice cube trays so that you can defrost as much or as little as you want at any one time. Simply spoon the mixture into ice cube trays and freeze flat for a couple of hours, then pop out the cubes, transfer to a labelled freezer bag, and return to the freezer for up to 3 months.

TO COOK FROM FROZEN: The cubes of pesto will defrost really quickly when added to a hot pan, simply add as many as you need and cook, stirring until defrosted, then use as described in the *To Use* section, left.

RED PESTO

PREP: 5 MINUTES
**MAKES ABOUT 1 CUP
(240ML)**

1 tsp frozen, chopped garlic
2 tsp frozen, chopped red
  chillies
¼ cup (35g) pine nuts
1 large jar (270g drained
  weight) semi-dried
  tomatoes in oil, drained
½ cup (120ml) olive oil
  (you can use the oil from
  the drained jar)
handful of flat leaf parsley
½ teaspoon of salt

01 Simply transfer all of the ingredients to a
blender and blend to your desired consistency
– depending on if you prefer a coarser or
smoother pesto. If the mixture is too dry,
simply add a little more oil.

TO USE: The pesto is now
ready to use. It is delicious used
to dress pasta or spooned over
grilled fish or meats.

TO FREEZE: I like to freeze
pesto in ice cube trays so that
you can defrost as much or as
little as you want at any one
time. Simply spoon the mixture
into ice cube trays and freeze
flat for a couple of hours, then
pop out the cubes, transfer to a
labelled freezer bag, and return
to the freezer for up to
3 months.

TO COOK FROM FROZEN:
The cubes of pesto will defrost
really quickly when added to a
hot pan, simply add as many as
you need and cook, stirring until
defrosted, then use as described
in the *To Use* section, left.

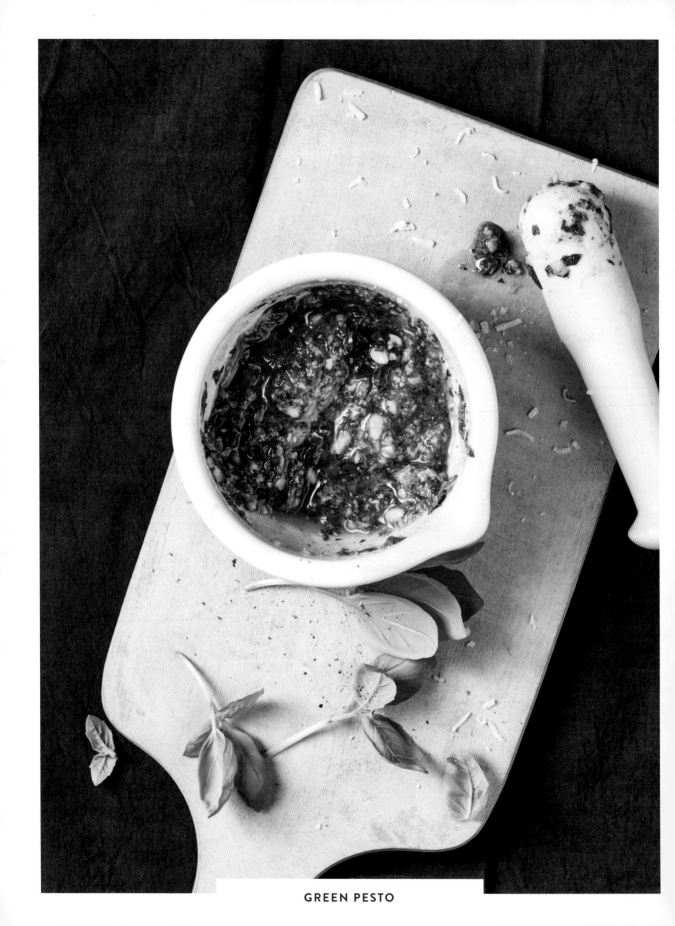

GREEN PESTO

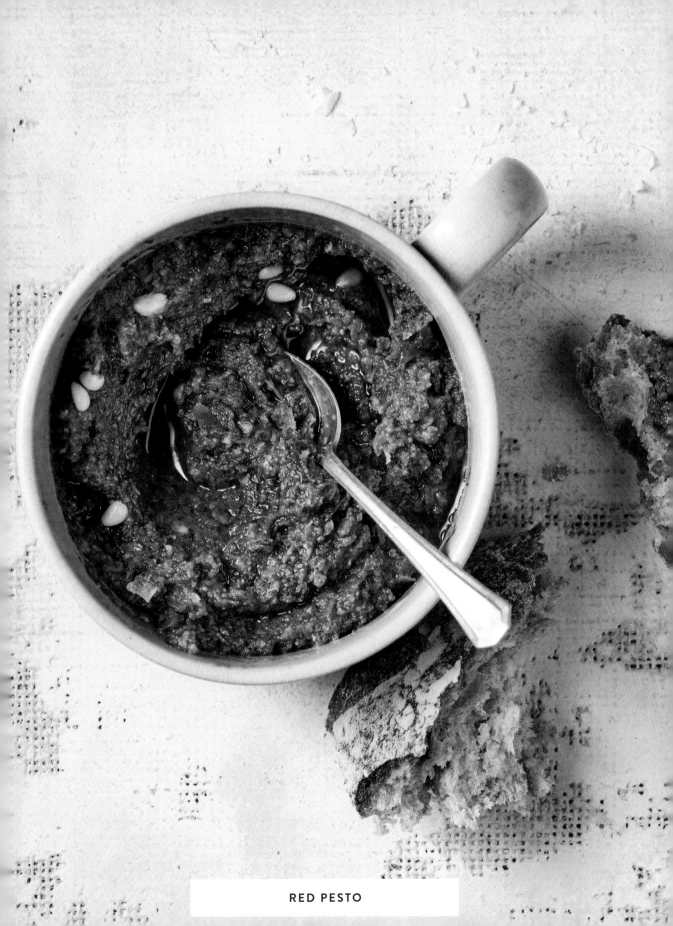

RED PESTO

THREE WAYS WITH...

PESTO

Now that you've prepared your Pesto, what are you going to do with it? Below are three simple ideas for different ways of serving it that will keep mealtimes feeling fresh and different every time.

PESTO-TOPPED MONKFISH WITH PANCETTA

1 x 500g bag baby or new
   potatoes
½ cup (120ml) Green or Red
   Pesto (p.220 and 221)
4 monkfish fillets
   (about 200g each)
8 slices pancetta
splash of olive oil
greens of your choice, to serve
   (green beans, spinach or
   winter greens all work well)

01 Put the potatoes in a large pan, cover with water and bring to a boil over a medium heat, then reduce to a simmer and leave to cook for 20 minutes, until tender.

02 Meanwhile, spoon the pesto over the top of the monkfish fillets, then wrap each fillet in two slices of pancetta.

03 Heat a splash of olive oil in an ovenproof frying pan over a medium heat, then add the wrapped monkfish and pan-fry until crisp on all sides. Transfer to the oven for 10 minutes, to finish cooking.

04 While the monkfish is in the oven, cook your greens, then drain the potatoes and slice them into rounds. Divide the potatoes between serving plates, then spoon the cooked greens on top. Place a cooked monkfish fillet on each serving plate and serve hot.

PESTO PASTA WITH BACON

3 cups (270g) dried pasta of
  your choice (penne, farfalle or
  conchigliette work well)
splash of olive oil
1 cup (225g) bacon lardons
1 cup (240ml) Green or Red
  Pesto (p.220 and 221)
salad, to serve

01 Bring a large pan of water to the boil, then
    add the pasta and cook for 10–12 minutes,
    until tender.
02 Heat the olive oil in a frying pan over a
    medium heat, then add the bacon and cook,
    stirring occasionally, until crisp and golden.
03 Drain and rinse the pasta through a colander.
    Add the pasta back to the pan along with
    the pesto and return to the heat to heat the
    pesto. Add the bacon and stir to combine.
    Divide the pasta between serving plates and
    serve warm with the salad alongside.

PESTO PIZZA WITH VINE TOMATOES, ROCKET & GOAT'S CHEESE

1 x shop-bought, ready-rolled
  pizza dough
½–1 cup (120–240ml) Green
  or Red Pesto (p.220 and 221)
10 cherry tomatoes, halved
125g goat's cheese
2 handfuls rocket

01 Preheat the oven to 180°C/350°F/gas mark 4
    and line a baking tray with greaseproof paper.
02 Unroll the pizza base and set on the prepared
    baking tray, then spread the pesto over the
    top. Scatter over the tomatoes and crumble
    over the goat's cheese.
03 Transfer to the oven and cook for 15–20
    minutes, until golden and bubbling and the
    base is crisp. Remove from the oven and
    garnish with a couple of handfuls of rocket,
    then slice and serve.

DESSERTS

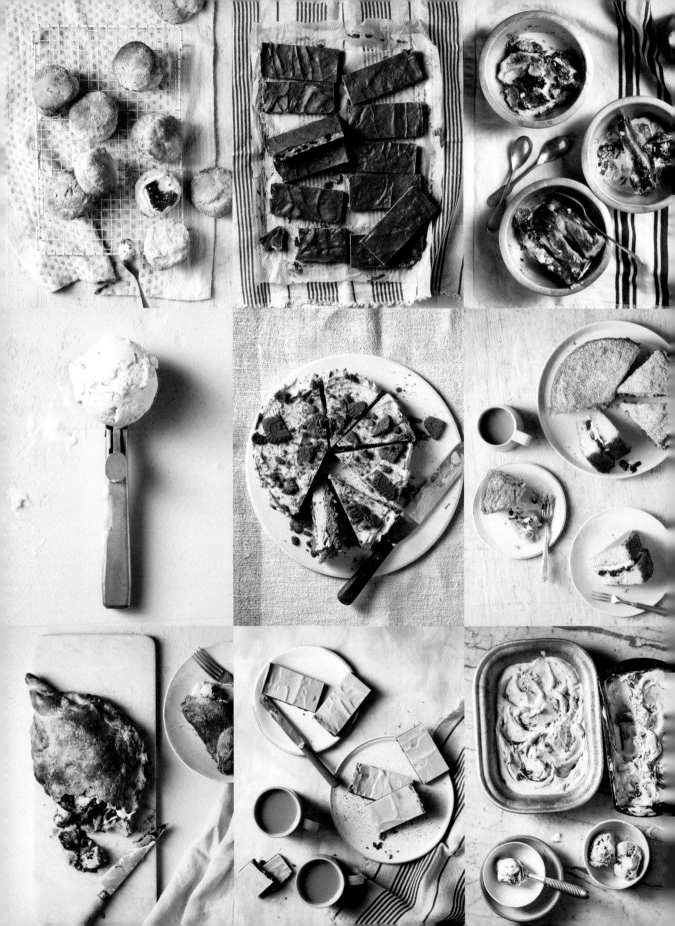

DESSERTS

When I need to de-stress, I bake a cake. Filling my kitchen with sweet smells and knowing that I will soon have a delicious treat for my family to eat makes this my favourite kind of cooking. Batching baked goods and desserts means that I've always got something sweet to offer visitors and putting most of it in the freezer as I cook it saves me from eating it myself!

In this chapter you'll find simple, delicious recipes for all my favourite sweet treats, from a showstopping but deceptively simple Biscoff Cheesecake or tempting Ice Cream Cookies to a classic Victoria Sponge. All of the recipes freeze brilliantly and can be whipped out whenever you have guests or just feel the need for something sweet.

VICTORIA SANDWICH

PREP: 15 MINUTES
COOK: 25 MINUTES
MAKES ONE 20CM (8IN) CAKE, SERVING 8

250g margarine
1½ cups (250g) caster sugar
1 tsp vanilla extract
1¾ cups (250g) self-raising flour
2 tsp baking powder
4 large eggs
To Serve:
jam of your choice
lightly whipped cream
icing sugar, to dust

I must admit to being a fan of packet mix when making chocolate cake, as the result is always deliciously moist, but for vanilla cake I have never found anything as good as traditional, homemade Victoria Sandwich.

This recipe and the Scones use many of the same ingredients, so I simply weigh out the ingredients for both recipes in separate bowls, then make the recipes side-by-side.

01 Preheat the oven to 190°C/375°F/gas mark 5 and grease and line two 20cm (8in) cake tins. For speed, you can use cake liners for this.

02 In a large bowl, cream together the margarine, caster sugar and vanilla extract with an electric whisk until light and fluffy.

03 In a separate bowl, combine the flour and baking powder. Beat one of the eggs into the butter mixture, then sift in a little of the flour and mix to combine. Continue adding the flour and eggs in this way until they are all incorporated.

04 Divide the mixture between the two cake tins, levelling it out with a spatula or palette knife, then transfer to the oven for 20–25 minutes, until golden brown, well risen and an inserted skewer comes out clean.

While the cakes are in the oven, make the scones.

05 Leave in the tins to cool slightly, then turn out onto a wire rack and set aside to cool to room temperature.

TO SERVE: Once the cakes have cooled to room temperature, spread one half with a generous coating of jam and top with whipped cream. Place the other cake on top, then dust with icing sugar, slice and serve.

TO FREEZE: Once the cakes have cooled to room temperature, wrap each half in clingfilm, then transfer to a labelled freezer bag and freeze flat for up to 3 months.

TO SERVE FROM FROZEN: Remove from the freezer and set aside to defrost – this should only take about 2 hours. Once defrosted, assemble and serve the cake as described in the *To Serve* section, left.

SCONES

PREP: 10 MINUTES
COOK: 12 MINUTES
MAKES 10

2 cups (220g) self-raising
  flour
3 tsp baking powder
pinch of salt
6 tablespoons (85g)
  unsalted butter
¼ cup (50g) caster sugar
1 egg, beaten
⅔ cup (160ml) milk
To Serve:
jam of your choice
clotted or lightly whipped
  cream

01 Sift the flour and baking powder into a large bowl, then add the salt, butter and sugar and use your fingers to rub the butter into the dry ingredients until you reach a breadcrumb consistency.

02 Add the egg, then pour in the milk a little at a time, stirring between additions, until the dough comes together. The dough should be sticky but not so wet that it doesn't hold its shape.

03 Turn the dough out onto a lightly floured surface and flatten to a rough round around 2.5cm (1in) thick. Using a 5.5cm (2¼in) cutter, stamp out rounds of the dough, rerolling the scraps as necessary. There should be enough dough for 10 scones.

TO COOK: Place the scones on a lined baking tray and transfer to an oven preheated to 220°C/425°F/gas mark 7 for 10–12 minutes, until golden and well risen. Leave to cool, then serve spread with jam and cream.

TO FREEZE: Place the uncooked scones on a lined baking tray and transfer to the freezer to freeze for 3–4 hours, then transfer to a labelled freezer bag and freeze flat for up to 3 months.

TO COOK FROM FROZEN: These can be cooked directly from frozen. Simply, place the scones on a lined baking tray and transfer to an oven preheated to 220°C/425°F/ gas mark 7 for 15 minutes, then served as described in the *To Cook* section, left.

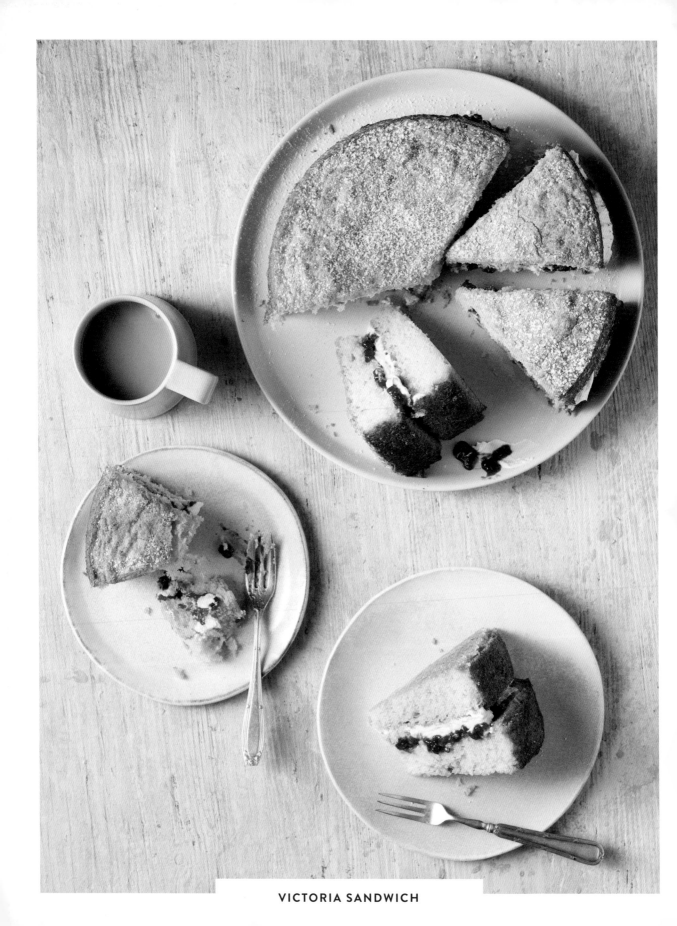

VICTORIA SANDWICH

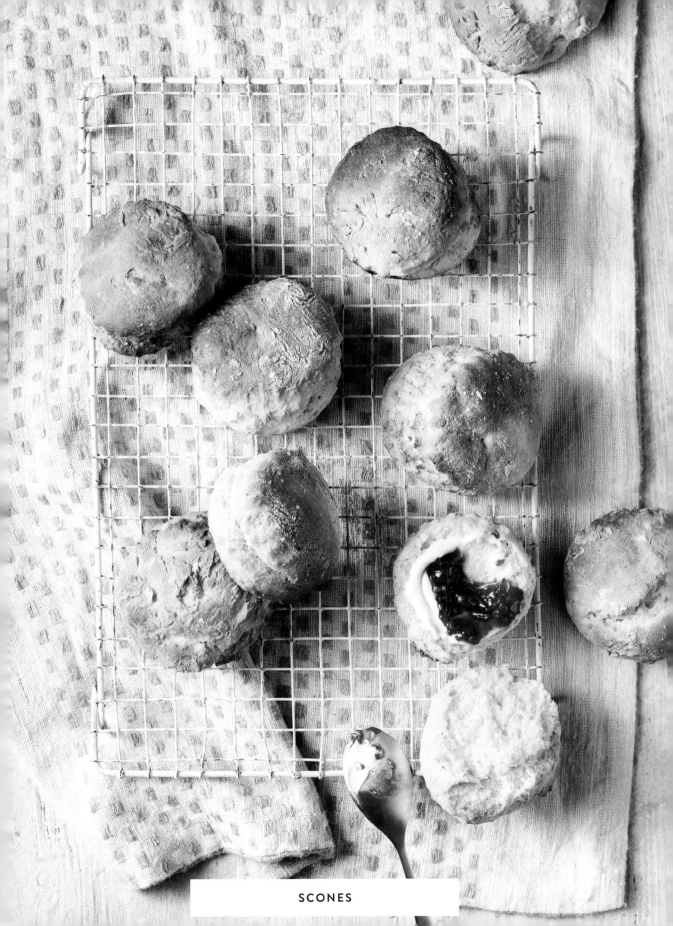

SCONES

CHOCOLATE RAISIN SLICES

PREP: 20 MINUTES, PLUS CHILLING
MAKES 12 LARGE OR 24 SMALL PIECES

300g rich tea biscuits
125g butter, cut into small cubes
1 cup (240ml) sweetened condensed milk
scant 1½ cups (200g) raisins
180g milk chocolate, broken into pieces

From school bake sales to charity coffee mornings, there are always times when you are expected to rustle up a yummy homemade treat at the drop of a hat. These moreish treats can be kept in the freezer, ready to whip out and impress anyone that comes knocking.

01 Grease a 35 x 25cm (14 x 10in) baking tray and line with greaseproof paper.

02 Put the biscuits in a food processor and process to a fine rubble. Alternatively, put them in a freezer bag and seal, ensuring that you remove any air, then bash with a rolling pin to crush.

> If you are also making the Peppermint Slices, crush the biscuits and mint chocolate in the same food processor now, then continue to work through both recipes side-by-side.

03 Place a large saucepan o-ver a low heat, then add the butter and condensed milk and stir until melted and well combined.

04 Add the crushed biscuits to the pan along with the raisins, then stir together until well combined. Pour the mixture into your prepared tray, pressing it down to a flat, even layer. Set aside.

05 Place the chocolate in a heat-proof bowl over a pan of barely simmering water and stir until melted. Pour the chocolate over the mixture in the tin and use a palette knife to create a thin, even layer covering the top of the Raisin Slice. Transfer to the fridge for 2–3 hours, until the mixture has firmed up and the chocolate has fully set.

06 Remove from the fridge and set aside for 20 minutes or so to allow the chocolate to soften slightly, then slice into pieces of your desired size.

TO SERVE: The slices are now ready to serve and can be kept in an airtight container for up to a week.

TO FREEZE: This can be frozen unsliced in the baking tray or as individual slices. Either way, simply wrap with clingfilm, transfer to a labelled freezer bag and freeze flat.

TO SERVE FROM FROZEN: Simply remove from the freezer and set aside until fully defrosted. Individual slices will defrost in a couple of hours, larger pieces will take a little longer.

PEPPERMINT SLICES

PREP: 20 MINUTES,
PLUS CHILLING
**MAKES 12 LARGE OR
24 SMALL PIECES**

300g rich tea biscuits
80g mint chocolate sticks
  (I use Matchmakers)
100g butter, cut into small
  cubes
1 x 397g can sweetened
  condensed milk
1 x 200g bar mint
  chocolate, broken into
  pieces
½ tsp peppermint essence
150g white chocolate,
  broken into pieces
3 drops green food
  colouring (optional)

01 Grease a 35 x 25cm (14 x 10in) baking tray and line with
    greaseproof paper.
02 Put the biscuits and mint chocolate sticks in a food processor
    and process to a fine rubble. Alternatively, put them in a freezer
    bag and seal, ensuring that you remove any air as you do so,
    then bash with a rolling pin to reach the same consistency.
03 Place a large saucepan over a low heat, add the butter,
    condensed milk and mint chocolate and stir until melted, then
    add the peppermint essence and stir again until well combined.
04 Add the crushed biscuits to the pan and stir until well
    combined, then pour the mixture into the prepared baking tray
    and press down to a flat, even layer. Set aside.
05 Place the white chocolate in a heat-proof bowl over a pan of
    barely simmering water and stir until melted, then stir in the
    green food colouring, if using. Pour the chocolate over the
    mixture in the tin and use a palette knife to create a thin, even
    layer covering the top of the Peppermint Slice. Transfer to the
    fridge for 2–3 hours, until the mixture has firmed up and the
    chocolate has fully set.
06 Remove from the fridge and set aside for 20 minutes or so to
    allow the chocolate to soften slightly, then slice into pieces of
    your desired size.

TO SERVE: The slices are now ready to serve and can be kept in an airtight container for up to a week.

TO FREEZE: This can be frozen unsliced in the baking tray or as individual slices. Either way, simply wrap with clingfilm, transfer to a labelled freezer bag and freeze flat.

TO SERVE FROM FROZEN: Simply remove from the freezer and set aside until fully defrosted. Individual slices will defrost in a couple of hours, larger pieces will take a little longer.

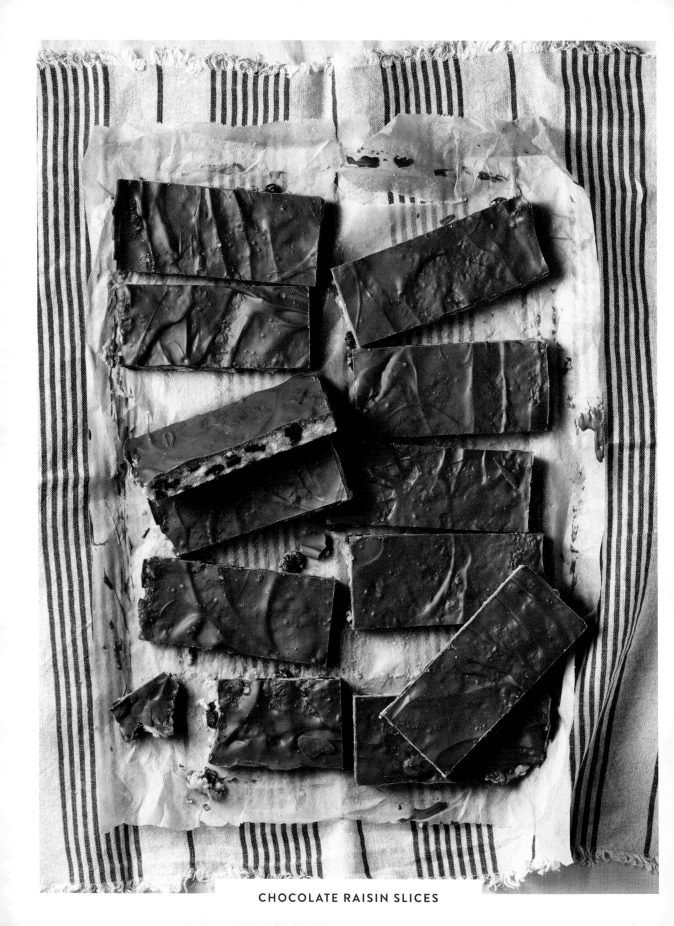

CHOCOLATE RAISIN SLICES

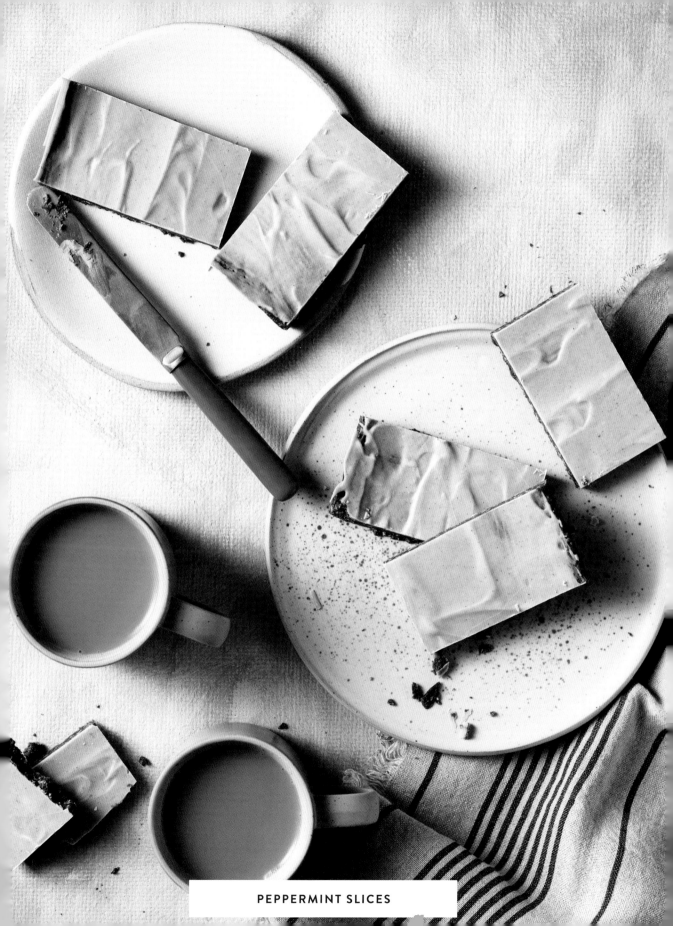

PEPPERMINT SLICES

ICE CREAM COOKIES

PREP: 15 MINUTES
COOK: 14 MINUTES
SERVES 4

1 cup (225g) soft, unsalted butter
1 cup (200g) soft brown sugar
1 tsp vanilla extract
3 eggs
1½ cups (145g) rolled oats
¼ cup (40g) chocolate chips
2 cups (260g) self-raising flour
1 x quantity vanilla ice cream (p.239) or store-bought vanilla ice cream, to serve

Having a batch of cookie dough ready to go in the freezer means that you're only ever 15 minutes away from fresh cookies, which can only be a good thing! Make the cookies as they are, or sandwich them together with vanilla ice cream, as below, for an extra special treat. Note that the cookies need to be fully frozen before baking, so you will need to get the dough in the freezer the day before you want to serve them.

01 In a large bowl, cream the softened butter and sugar with an electric whisk until light and airy. Add the vanilla extract, then add the eggs one at a time, beating between each addition, until well combined.

02 Add the oats and chocolate to the mix and sift in the flour, then whisk again until the mixture has come together to form a soft dough.

03 Lay a large, rectangular sheet of greaseproof paper on the countertop and tip the cookie dough out onto it. Fold the greaseproof around the dough, then use it to roll the dough into a cylinder shape around 5cm (2in) in diameter. Fold over the ends of the greaseproof paper, then secure the whole thing with tape. Transfer to the freezer and freeze flat overnight or until needed.

TO COOK FROM FROZEN: Remove the dough from the freezer and unroll the greaseproof paper. Using a hot knife, cut 1cm- (½in-) thick rounds of the dough, returning any dough that you don't need to the freezer for later. Lay the cookie-dough rounds on a lined baking sheet, leaving space for the cookies to spread between each one, then bake in an oven preheated to 180°C/350°F/gas mark 4 for 12–14 minutes, until golden and firm. Leave to cool on the trays for a couple of minutes, then transfer to a cooling rack to cool completely.

TO SERVE: Once cooled, use the cookies to sandwich scoops of vanilla ice cream, then neaten up the edges with a palette knife or spatula. Serve quickly, before the ice cream starts to melt.

VANILLA ICE CREAM

D

PREP: 5 MINUTES, PLUS
FREEZING
SERVES 4

1 x 600ml pot double
   cream
1 x 397g can sweetened
   condensed milk
1 tsp vanilla extract

01 Put the double cream, condensed milk and vanilla extract in a large bowl and stir gently to just combine, then, using an electric whisk, whisk the mixture until thick, about 5 minutes.

02 Transfer the mixture to a freezer proof dish and cover with a lid or a layer of clingfilm followed by a layer of foil. Transfer to the freezer until completely set.

Note
If you want to be really organized, once the ice cream is completely set, transfer individual scoops to a freezer bag and return to the freezer. Then simply remove the scoops from the freezer as you need them.

TO SERVE FROM FROZEN:
Once set, the ice cream can be served immediately.

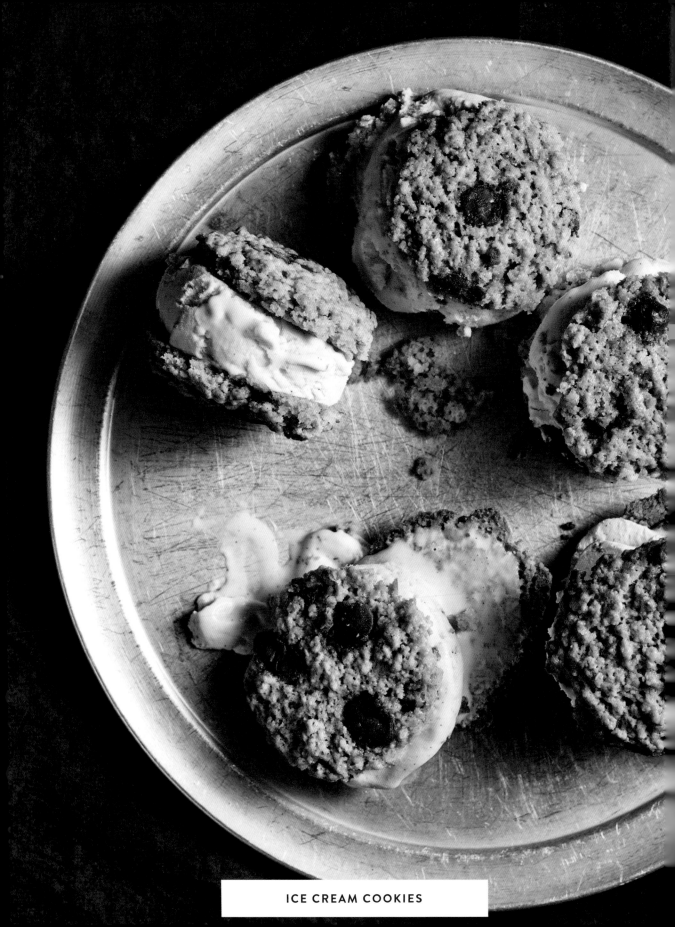

ICE CREAM COOKIES

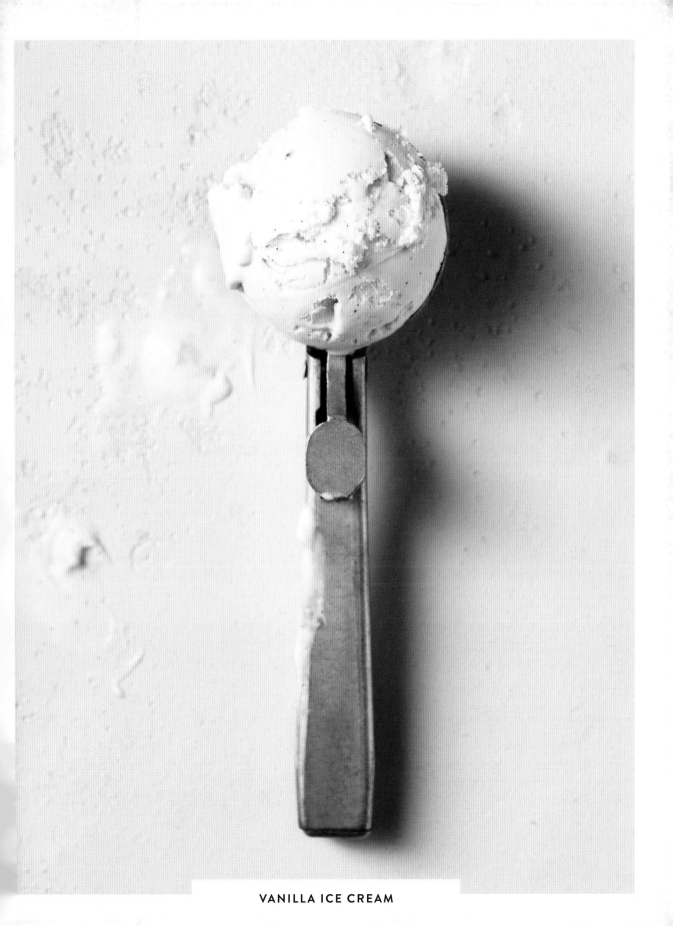

VANILLA ICE CREAM

FROZEN BISCOFF CHEESECAKE

PREP: 30 MINS, PLUS FREEZING

MAKES ONE 20CM (8IN) CHEESECAKE, SERVING 6–8

2 cups (75g) honey and nut corn flakes

1 x 400g jar smooth caramelized biscuit spread (I use Biscoff)

270g cream cheese

butter, for greasing

3–4 caramel flavoured biscuits, crushed, to decorate (optional)

This cheesecake always goes down a treat and is best eaten when slightly frozen, making it perfect for preparing ahead! This would also be lovely made with chocolate hazelnut spread, rather than biscuit, so feel free to substitute the ingredients to suit your tastes.

01 Grease a 20cm (8in) loose-bottomed flan tin with butter.

02 Put the honey and nut corn flakes in a bowl with one third of the caramelized biscuit spread and mix together to combine, then press into the base of the prepared tin in a flat, even layer. Transfer to the fridge to set for 20 minutes while you prepare the topping.

03 Put the cream cheese and remaining caramelized biscuit spread in a large bowl and beat together until well combined. The mixture should be a uniformly 'biscuity' colour with no visible flecks of cream cheese. Set aside.

> If you are also making the Biscoff Ice Cream, do this now while you are waiting for the cheesecake base to set.

04 After 20 minutes, remove the cheesecake base from the fridge and spoon the cream cheese mixture over it, pressing down into the tin and levelling with a palette knife or spatula to create an even, level topping. Scatter over the crushed caramel biscuits to decorate.

TO FREEZE: The cheesecake needs to set in the freezer before serving. Set on a flat baking tray and transfer to the freezer for 24 hours, then cover in a layer of clingfilm followed by a layer of foil and return to the freezer for up to 1 month.

TO SERVE FROM FROZEN: This cheesecake is best eaten still slightly frozen. Simply remove from the freezer and cut into portions, then leave for 15–20 minutes to thaw slightly before serving. Return the remaining cheesecake to freezer.

BISCOFF ICE CREAM

PREP: 10 MINS
MAKES APPROX.
1 LITRE

1 x 600ml pot double
    cream
1 x 397g can sweetened
    condensed milk
1 tsp vanilla extract
200g (½ a jar) of crunchy
    caramelized biscuit spread
    (I use Biscoff)

I use Biscoff crunchy spread for this. If you can only find the smooth variety, the ice cream will still be delicious but, if you are looking for that extra crunch, you could crumble over a couple of biscuits before serving.

01 Put the double cream, condensed milk and vanilla extract in a large bowl and stir gently to just combine, then, using an electric whisk, beat the mixture until thick, about 5 minutes.

02 Spoon dollops of the biscuit spread over, then use a palette knife to ripple it through the ice cream.

03 Transfer the mixture to a freezer proof dish and cover with a lid or a layer of clingfilm followed by a layer of foil. Transfer to the freezer until completely set.

If you are also making the Biscoff Cheesecake, return to step 4 now.

Note
If you want to be really organized, once the ice cream is completely set, transfer individual scoops to a freezer bag and return to the freezer. Then simply remove the scoops from the freezer as you need them.

TO SERVE FROM FROZEN:
Once frozen, the ice cream can be served immediately.

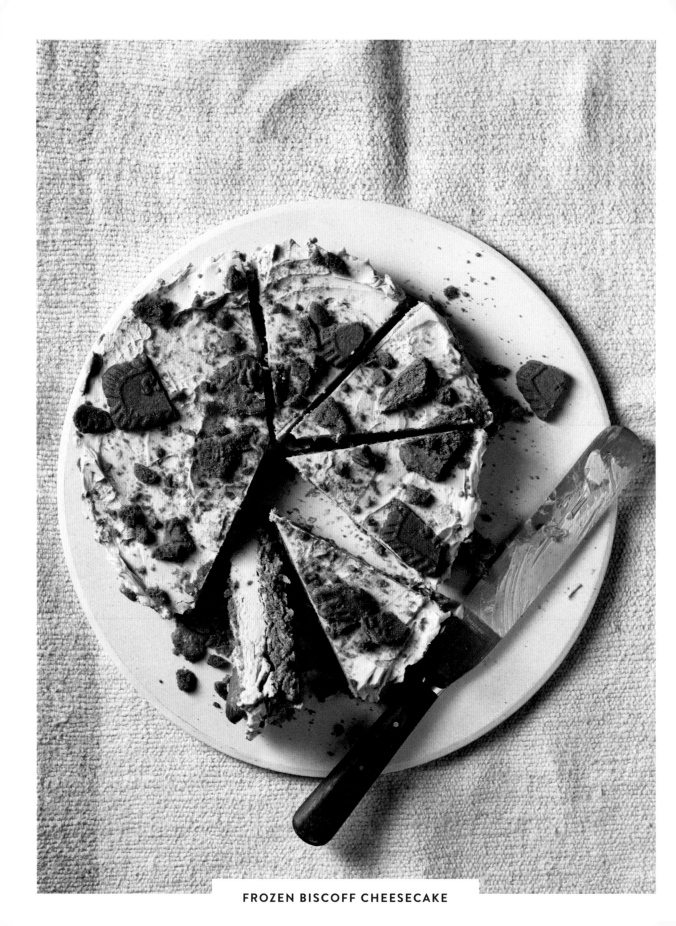

FROZEN BISCOFF CHEESECAKE

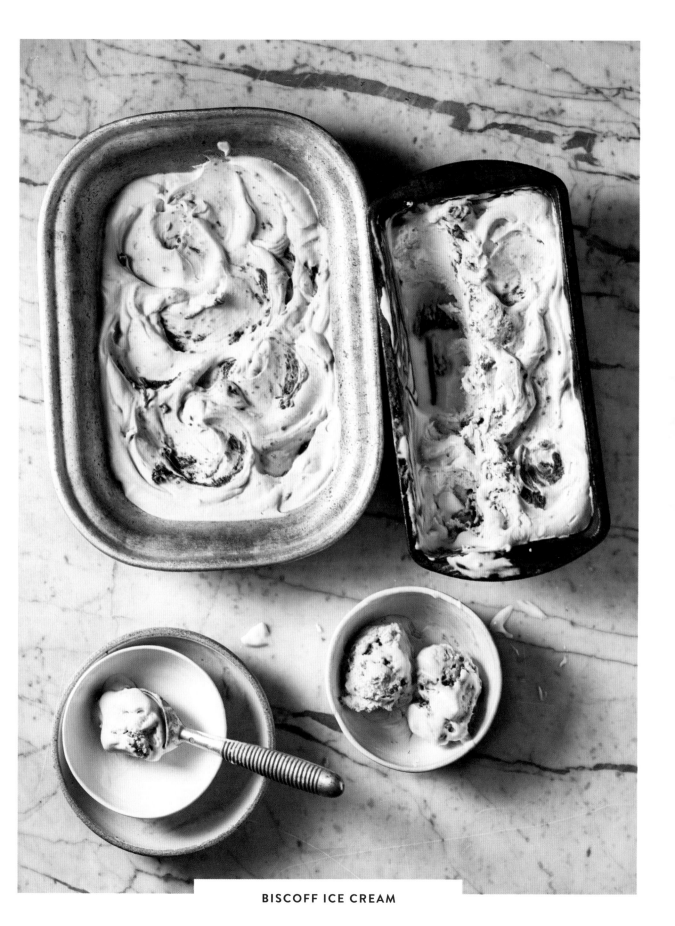

BISCOFF ICE CREAM

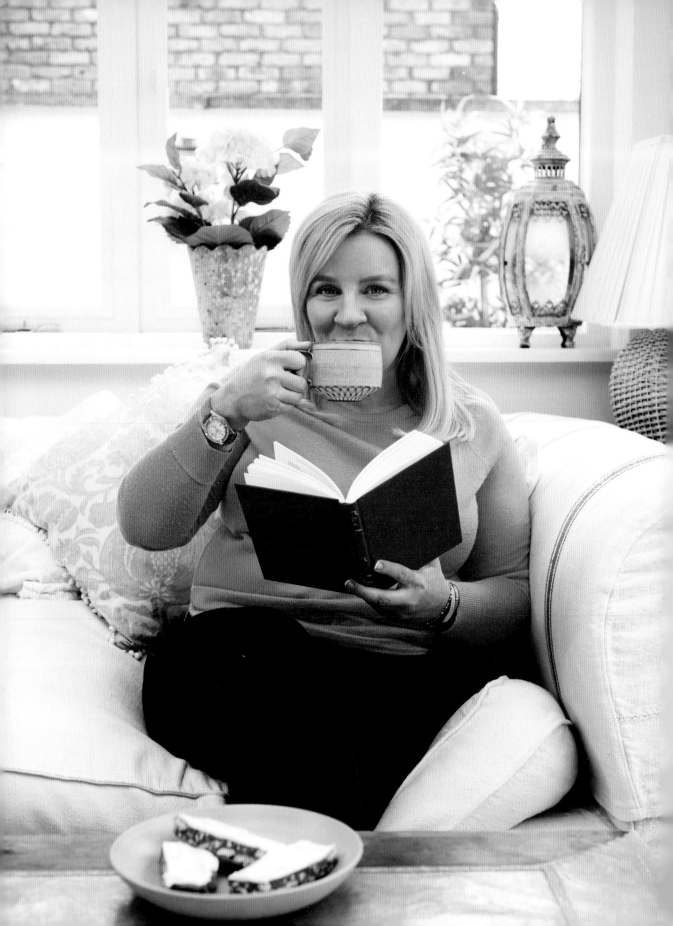

GOODBYE

So you've reached the end of my book – and I hope you've found plenty of tips, tricks and recipes to save time and money while you keep your freezer stocked, and your belly full.

But that's not the end of the batching journey. It's just the beginning! The recipes in this book are just a starting point, and when you've got the hang of the Batch Method, you can start to apply it to your own favourite recipes too. In no time at all, you may find you're approaching other household tasks in the same way, too.

Don't worry if you haven't switched on to the batching mentality overnight. It will come, little by little, as you start to think about this way of preparing and grouping your favourite meals by ingredient. I hope you get to make the most of the time you save, whether that's a cup of tea and a good book, or more time spent with friends and family rather than in the kitchen at mealtimes.

For more meal ideas and batching tips, or even to share your own batching success stories with me, you can find me at:

thebatchlady.com
facebook.com/thebatchlady
twitter.com/thebatchlady
instagram.com/thebatchlady

Believe in the batch!

Suzanne

INDEX

Q

ACKNOWLEDGEMENTS

If someone had told me two years ago that I would soon be writing a cookery book, I would have told them they were mad – yet here it is! It would not have happened without the wonderful group of friends who gathered in my kitchen for my first ever charity batch-cooking demonstration and encouraged me to do something more with it – to you guys I will be forever grateful. I'm so immensely thankful to everyone who has ever followed me on social media, visited my website, tried my recipes and spread the word. It was your amazing following that helped me get published, and without you guys this book wouldn't have happened ... you guys ROCK!

I would like to give my sincere thanks to Lisa Milton, Kate Fox and the rest of the team at Harper Collins for believing in The Batch Lady approach and for inviting me to write a book with them. It's been a fantastic journey and wonderful to work with so many great people. In particular Daniel Hurst, my project editor, and Georgina Hewitt, my designer, who spent many dedicated hours on the text and layout of the book – 10 Meals in 1 Hour was a huge challenge to fit into a recipe book and you guys made it look amazing! Danielle Wood for the fabulous photography and the fun times in the studio. She was ably assisted by Charlie Goodge, James Lee and Rosie Alsop, and I would like to thank them and also Ted Allen who retouched all of the images.

Thank you to Rosie Ramsden who created and styled the delicious food for photography with assistance from Kitty Coles and Rosie French – I never knew my recipes could look so stylish!

A huge shout out goes to Cathryn Summerhayes, my agent at Curtis Brown – I am so grateful for her continued guidance and advice which keeps me steering in the right direction. I also owe a massive thank you to my friend Harry, who was instrumental in getting me in front of agents and producers in London – your help will never be forgotten.

To Rebecca, thank you for all your admin help in getting me to this stage, and to Tara for those early photographs that helped me get started and looked so professional. Thank you also to my fab recipe testers, Victoria T, Tara, Julie, Lucy and Victoria L. The fact these recipes work so well is thanks to all your testing and help.

Most of all, I could not have done this without the love and support of my husband Peter and my two children Jake and Zara. Thank you for helping me through all the writing, filming, recipe testing, IT glitches, late nights, trips to cookery demonstrations, eating of the food and for putting up with the car smelling of fish for a week the time I locked my keys in it on the way back from the supermarket ... It's been a fab roller coaster ride and I'm so glad that you were all on it with me!

Suzanne